Ron Garner, BEd, MSc, is a health researcher, educator, author and speaker. Since his retirement he has devoted his life to discovering how we can live free from disease. Ron presents complex subjects in an organized, easy-to-understand manner. He is the author of the award-wining book, *Conscious Health* and lives in British Columbia, Canada.

THE DISEASE-FREE

REVOLUTION

Ron Garner

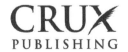

First published in the United Kingdom in 2014 by Crux Publishing Ltd.

ISBN: 978-1-909979-09-3
Copyright © Ron Garner, 2014

ISBN-13: 978-1-909979-09-3

Also available as an ebook:
eISBN: 978-1-909979-07-9

Requests for permission to reproduce material from this work should be sent
to hello@cruxpublishing.co.uk

www.cruxpublishing.co.uk

DISCLAIMER

Although the author has extensively researched sources to ensure the accuracy and completeness of the information contained in this book, no responsibility is assumed for errors, inaccuracies, or omissions, or inconsistencies herein. Any slights of people or organizations are unintentional. Neither the author nor the publisher is engaged in rendering professional advice or services to the individual reader. This book is not intended to be and should not be considered as a replacement for consultation, diagnosis, or treatment by a doctor or licensed healthcare practitioner. Please consult your personal physician or healthcare practitioner before starting any diet, taking non-prescription supplements, or beginning any new health treatment. The intent of this book is only to offer information to help you cooperate with your healthcare practitioner in your mutual search for health. Neither the author nor the publisher shall be liable or responsible for any loss or damage allegedly arising from any information or any suggestions in this book.

While the author has made every effort to provide accurate Internet addresses at the time of publication, neither the publisher nor author assumes any responsibility for errors or for changes that occur after publication. Further, the publisher does not have control over and does assume any responsibility for author or third-party websites or their content.

CONTENTS

INTRODUCTION

Why a Revolution?

In my firmly held opinion that is exactly what we need, because we are being deceived and lied to on a regular basis by the very people and industries we have been taught to rely on for our health and nutritional well-being. That's why I wrote this book – to help you and people like you. This book will explain how our acceptance of, and reliance on, present medical practices and commercially-produced food with chemical additives are making millions of people sick. You see, we are part of an industry. It is called the sickness or disease industry, and we are the market. As long as people continue to be uninformed and confused, and don't take some responsibility for their own health, the sickness money-industry just keeps getting bigger and bigger. All the while, we keep getting sicker and sicker – suffering, losing quality and joy of life, and dying much sooner than we need to.

The only ones who can escape this present-day sickness trap are those who take responsibility for their own health by learning how their bodies are designed to operate, and then help their bodies to build health and really enjoy life.

That's what this *Disease-Free Revolution* book is all about – giving you the keys you need to unlock the door to see through the sickness illusions. Great health and freedom from disease can be yours. You just have to want them badly enough to work for them and be prepared to change some things in your life to achieve the health you were meant to have.

When you have good health, everything is possible. Without health, nothing matters. If we have lost our health and then regained it, life becomes enjoyable and exciting again. New possibilities can open up. We don't have to deteriorate with age as we see happening to many people all around us.

Our mind is where we should begin the process of making changes in our lives. We must be willing to view life and ourselves in new ways to recover from a disease process. This takes courage, but a sincere desire for change allows this to happen.

Welcome to the Disease-Free Revolution program

At the time of writing this book I am 76 years old and enjoying some of the best health of my life, but it hasn't always been that way. I'd like to tell you a little about what brought me to research natural health, which then led me to develop what you are about to read in this *Disease-Free Revolution* program.

In my 50s, my health was going downhill and I lost faith in the drug-only approach. After many years of following it I wasn't getting better, so it no longer made sense to me. There had to be a better way. Ultimately I found it to be nature's way. It took me a lot of time and effort to sort through all the confusing points of view about health. But as I kept researching I learned more. And during this time I changed my eating habits and worked on detoxifying my body.

I read all the books and research papers I could find to learn about how our bodies work and how different foods affect them. I sought out and learned from all the successful alternative and natural health teachers I could discover. Men like Dr. Joel Robbins at the College of Natural Health in Tulsa Oklahoma; Dr. Michael O'Brien, a former medical doctor, who was told by other doctors that he would die from cancer and liver disease, but who cured himself and then turned away from his medical practice to teach people about natural health; Dr. Bernard Jensen, a naturopathic doctor who had 60 years of clinical practice and wrote some 55 books on nutrition, detoxification, and natural health; Dr. Francis Pottenger, who in the 1930s conducted nutritional experiments with 900 cats to learn the difference between a diet of raw or cooked food; Dr. M. T. Morter, a chiropractor from whom I learned how the acid/alkaline balance in the body works; Dr. Nicholas Gonzales, a successful alternative cancer doctor; Dr. Jerry Tennant of Irving Texas, who is a foremost authority on the electrical nature of the human body; and Douglas Wyatt, who is considered to be the father of bovine colostrum. There are many others, but these are some of the prominent teachers who I am proud to call my mentors.

During my learning process, I experimented with everything I thought might contribute to a good health program. I made mistakes along the way but kept at it, and after a while I started to see results. My energy came back, the foggy mind feeling I had went away and I could think clearly again, allergies became fewer and less severe, asthma started to disappear, skin problems began to clear, chronic indigestion and diarrhea ceased, and my sleep became more restful and longer.

I continue to work on eating properly and helping my body to detoxify as it goes through its occasional but necessary brief episodes of healing, which I will talk more about in a later chapter on how the body heals. Now, in my mid 70s I feel wonderful and I look and feel younger than my age. For me, life is joyful and exciting again. In the next chapter I'll tell you about my personal health story in a bit more detail.

I'm telling my story and presenting this natural health program so that it might be an encouragement and plan for other people who are searching for better health answers in their lives. I hope it will be for you. I fully believe that it is possible to reverse degenerating health as I have done, and start to achieve the same health benefits I now enjoy.

I'm sure you realize that disease is really out of control in our western society. We are presented with the notion that it all happens by random chance, and that disease is inevitable as we grow older. Yes, some foods and behaviours are bad for us, but are we ever clear on just how bad, or what we can do about it? I think we need a fundamental change, a revolution really, in the way most people think about health and disease because our present situation simply isn't working. The disease situation in our society is getting worse. In my opinion, we need a radical change in the underlying beliefs we have been taught to accept because many of them are simply not true! We need change, and change always begins with a different or revolutionary way of thinking.

The knowledge I'm suggesting is nothing new – it's always been there. We used to eat whole natural foods, but in the last few generations big business has taken over and pushed natural ways aside. If products are mass produced and sit in warehouses, then shipped to retailers and finally arrive at your table months later, it seems only logical that a process like that requires preservatives as well as chemical enhancers to make them taste better. However, it is that very process that depletes vital nutrients and adds harmful chemicals. Good for business, not so good for health.

An almost total reliance on pharmaceutical drugs, while ignoring nutrition, has trapped us into treating only the symptoms of disease. There is very little, if any, actual healing or prevention of disease. We've turned the management of our own health over to others and stopped being our own decision-makers. That, I think, is the most important point where our personal health is concerned. *We* need to be in control and make decisions ourselves – in our own best interests. I'm not talking about dismissing all medicine. What I am talking about is the preventative maintenance and healing of your own body by giving it what it needs to heal and stay healthy – the way nature intended.

I have designed this Disease-Free Revolution program to answer many questions about why disease is out of control, and give you solutions to apply in your own life to correct or prevent health problems for yourself and your family members. It takes courage, independent thinking, and perseverance to walk a path that is different from what most others are taking in any society. We may not be able to change the world, but we can change ourselves and then be an inspiring example to others. As Mahatma Ghandi said:

"You need to be the change you wish to see in the world."

Where our health is concerned, it starts with your understanding how you can escape the present mindset of inevitable disease and temporary pharmaceutical fixes used to make you feel better, while not really healing the *causes* of why you are sick. Most of us should be able to change our lifestyles and move on to live disease-free well into our elder years.

I wrote *The Disease-Free Revolution* with exactly this intention in mind – to give you the knowledge and tools you need to be in control of your own health program. If you follow the guidelines I lay out for you, I truly believe that you can live in great health. I believe it's possible to live free of heart disease, cancer, joint pain, dementia, Alzheimer's, diabetes and all the other so-called 'normal' signs of aging in our society. But you know something? They aren't normal at all. And neither is being seriously overweight. These conditions have become commonplace to the point where most of us just accept them as being a natural part of aging. But I would like you to understand this – they are not a natural part of aging and you don't have to slide into these conditions. This *Disease-Free Revolution* book will show you how. The tools are here. You just have to learn them and use them.

In this program I have included everything you need to know about natural health, because that is the way your body works – naturally! Pharmaceutical drugs may save lives but they can't build health. Drugs may have a place in therapeutically treating a serious illness, but they should not be considered as long-term maintenance solutions because they do not correct illness causes or body deficiencies.

This natural health knowledge is powerful stuff. Don't underestimate it! The information here is easy to understand. There aren't any complicated and confusing explanations. And this course of knowledge is quite complete because it covers the physical, mental, and emotional areas that together form the connected parts of our health make-up. Furthermore, these principles will never go out of date. They will apply just as well for your great-grandchildren in future years as they will for you now.

CHAPTER 1

WHY WE GET SICK

WHY WE LOSE OUR HEALTH

As we age, why do most of us become sick and lose the healthy body we had when we were young? In simple terms, there are only two main reasons for losing your health:

1. Lack of knowledge – you just don't know why disease happens or how you can avoid it.

2. Lack of effort – you *know* that eating foods and drinking sweetened beverages that are not good for you are undermining your health, but you do it anyway. You think you don't have time, or you don't want to make the effort to do the things that will keep you healthy.

I can't do anything about the second reason, but this whole health program will take care of the first. It will give you the knowledge you might not have had before. That is, you will understand how your health is lost and how it can be won, and you will know how to do it.

Fat Storage

Knowing how to be healthy and not carrying extra pounds around on your body go hand in hand. A truly healthy body does not have extra fat because it doesn't need it! When your body is being fed nutritious food, it just gets on with the job of building a healthy body. Excessive fat storage is caused by eating too many of the wrong kind of calories and foods that are laced with chemicals. In this program you are going to learn what the right kinds of calories are and how you can get them into your diet.

Extra fat is where the body stores toxins it can't get rid of. And toxins, which are poisons to your body, are in most of the modern commercial foods we eat. So your body has no choice but to lay down fat as insulation to keep toxins away from your vital organs. And because there are too many of these wrong calories and chemical additives in the food it has to process, its organs of elimination become clogged. The cycle just keeps on going and adding up. When you start eating foods your body can use to build health and cleanse your body of toxins, the weight problem will take care of itself. It usually just falls off automatically. It is a bonus while you are getting healthier.

As you read through this program please keep in mind that while I am talking about how health is lost or won, I am also giving you the keys to how you can become healthy and permanently reach your ideal weight. There is no magic weight loss pill or diet that will also make you healthy and keep you from developing one or more of the many diseases we see all around us today.

The *Disease-Free Revolution* program way is the slower but permanent and continual weight loss and health solution. Truth and knowledge are your paths to power. But they only become power to you when you learn them and put them into practice.

In this program I'm going to tell you about:

- The time-tested truths concerning health and disease
- Why disease happens and how you can avoid it, or turn it around once symptoms start to appear
- Why we put on weight and can't seem to take it off permanently
- Why illnesses that seem to run in your family, called inherited disease conditions, don't need to happen to you
- Why your health is a partnership between you and your body, and why your body needs your cooperation
- Why, as a society, we are sick and getting sicker
- Why conventional health care is really just "sick-care" or "disease maintenance"
- What conventional health care is good at and what you can do better for yourself
- Everything you need to know to be able to take control and be your own primary health advisor.

In this chapter I am going to talk about:

- My own personal story of how I regained my health
- What Conscious Health is
- Whether we have health care or sick care from the conventional medical system
- What the research findings are for our present day

disease situation
- How we got this way without being aware of it or knowing what we can do about it
- How the Disease-Free Revolution health plan is do-able for you and how you can start with small steps.

Discovering how to turn my own deteriorating health around, and creating my own program to restore it, was the most interesting, exciting, and rewarding thing I have ever done in my life. And it can be for you too.

MY PERSONAL STORY

By the time I was 6 months old, my body was covered with eczema. At the age of four, my tonsils were removed in hopes that would help with the problem. Yes really! Looking back on this now it is hard to understand that thinking. However, the eczema continued and the itch was excruciating especially during the spring and summer. As a child I would scratch myself until the inflamed skin bled. I remember many times calling out to my mother in the middle of the night and she would heat water to soak the bed sheets off me where they had dried into my skin. I couldn't go swimming in the lake with other kids where I lived because my skin was so sensitive due to the eczema all over my legs and arms. I had to wear long sleeves and pants all the time. At about the age of eight the eczema on my hands was so bad it became infected, which led to blood poisoning that almost took my life. The eczema continued to plague me until I got into my new health program in my 60s.

In my teens and 20s I developed allergies along with digestive problems, serious hay fever, hives, and more itching. I became allergic to grass and tree pollens, tobacco smoke, some chemicals in household cleaners, and animal dander (similar to dandruff). After I had children of my own I felt terrible that I could not let them have a dog or a cat because I was so seriously allergic to them.

Although I had some mild asthma as a young child, asthma began to affect me far more regularly at the age of 25, to the extent that I had to carry an inhaler with me at all times. In my early 30s I became seriously allergic to eggs. In my 40s, bowel issues and chronic diarrhea became another thing I had to cope with. I could go on, but these problems became a constant part of my life and I began to wear down. I could see myself in the mirror – rapidly aging. In my 50s I had a challenging educational administrative job and during those years I would need to take a nap during my lunch hour just to recharge my energy to finish each day's work.

It was then when I realized that the conventional medical approach was not improving my health because it was getting worse. I was facing a bleak future if I continued down the pharmaceutical treatment path. That's when I became desperate and determined to find some answers of my own. I couldn't believe that our bodies had to slide into disease as we got older. That's when I turned to researching natural health solutions.

My own health program development process took me about 15 years of research as well as much trial and error. One of the mistakes I made was to go on a five-day water fast, during which time I lost some muscle mass that was very difficult for me to recover. I tried many different supplements. Some were effective for me and some were not. But that's how I learned. Unfortunately, I didn't have a program such as the one I am presenting to you that sorted out the good from the bad and the safe from the risky. At this point in my life, approximately 90% of the health problems I suffered from had been corrected, but the remaining improvements had to wait until I learned about the major cause of most disease conditions, which I will tell you about in Chapter 8.

You see, our bodies are not meant to slide into disease as we get older, but in our present society with mass-produced foods, chemicals, toxins, stress, and over-use of pharmaceutical drugs, that's the result. Hospitals are overwhelmed and many people are taking several drug medications every day. Most of these people are dependent on them, in spite of their side effects. The worst part is that people don't understand how their bodies lose the ability to stay healthy, or how they can help themselves return to health. They are not conscious of what undermines and what builds health. That's what this program is all about. For the great majority of people, there is a way out of disease and back to vibrant health.

WHAT IS CONSCIOUS HEALTH?

Conscious Health is about being aware of what you are doing, and how it is helping or hindering your body's ability to produce energetic health well into your senior years. It's really up to you. Health can be your choice.

THE WAR ON DISEASE

We are losing the war on disease in our society in spite of all the medical advances. But if we change our thinking and look at our health problems in another way, there is hope. You CAN transform your health. The first part of that is to understand some truths about the conventional medical system almost everyone relies on.

So let's take a look at our conventional medical system, and what the disease statistics are today.

Do we have Healthcare or is it really just Sick Care?

When I started to open my mind to look beyond our present system of health care, these are some of the questions I began asking myself:

- Why aren't we being told about effective ways to live disease-free so we can stay healthy and enjoy our lives?
- Why are so many people in our society sick?
- Why does almost one out of every two people get cancer?
- Why does one out of every four people in America die of heart disease?
- Why are so many diseases such as diabetes, Alzheimer's, lung problems and high blood pressure out of control?
- Why are so many people overweight?
- Why is mercury, which has been labelled the most toxic non-radioactive metal known to humans, still used in dental fillings?
- Why are fluorides, which have the same toxicity as lead, being put into the drinking water of so many of our communities?

- Why are more and more of our children getting diseases?
- Why doesn't the medical system understand what causes disease?

It appeared to me that the present system is all about sickness and not really about health. We are deceived into believing that conventional doctors are there to help us be healthy, when in reality they are there to make us feel better – at least temporarily. So I begin by asking you a question: "Do you go to the doctor to find out about how to be healthy and stay healthy, even when you are feeling well? Or do you go to the doctor only when you get sick?"

That's why I believe that the present system is not about healthcare. It is about 'sick care'. We now have more medical schools, doctors, and hospitals than ever before, but we are sicker than before and it's getting worse. Why? The reason is that conventional medical care treats only the *symptoms* of disease. True healthcare works to correct the *causes* of disease. But I *ask* you this: "If you don't know the cause of something, how can you fix it?"

True healthcare uses natural methods, detoxification, foods, and herbs. This kind of traditional care has been practiced since the beginning of civilization. Today's medical system, which is barely a century old, tries to treat disease with chemicals, surgery, and radiation technologies. And you know something – it is not the fault of the doctors either, because that is the way they have been taught and forced to practice.

Medical doctors are trained to look for disease, and then to use pharmaceutical drugs as their treatment of choice. They receive almost no instruction in medical school about the nutritional aspects of disease prevention. After leaving medical school, doctors receive their ongoing education about the effectiveness of new drugs from pharmaceutical company representatives, whose main objective is to convince doctors to sell their products. Big-pharma is really the one in control, and profits are a main objective. The original meaning of 'Doctor' is 'Teacher.' But, it appears that most conventional medical doctors have forgotten that calling. For the most part they have just become prescription-writers, or as Dr. Bruce Lipton, renowned cell biologist and author of *The Biology of Belief,* calls them 'pharmaceutical patsies.' When was the last time a medical doctor spent time talking to you about nutrition and how to be healthy?

Conventional medicine, with its drug-treatment mindset, typically views the human body only as a chemical entity. This thinking is 80 to 90 years out of date and is based on the view that the universe is just made up of matter. This completely ignores the electrical energy factors of health. Here is the important point – all living things have *living* chemistry. Drugs contain no life and are therefore incapable of rebuilding life. In fact, they are often harmful. Still, the pharmaceutical industry bombards the public via various media, urging people to "ask your doctor if this drug is right for you." Yet the same ads list multiple possible harmful side effects that might be experienced. Now I ask you, is something wrong with this picture?

However, don't think that I am entirely against all drugs. I admit that in cases of life-threatening emergency, drugs can save lives, as they did for me when I had blood poisoning at age eight. I owe my life to penicillin, but drugs should be a temporary measure to save our body while we get back to helping it to naturally detoxify, replenish its nutritional and energy reserves, and strengthen its immune system.

Now just in case you still have absolute faith in the conventional medical system and place your unquestioning trust in it, and don't mind being put on several drug medications as time goes by you may want to consider the following:

What has changed in our society?

As a society we are becoming sicker and our hospitals are over-loaded. But let's consider how this picture has changed over the years. In the 1800s doctors who observed native populations in Africa, Kashmir, and northern Canada reported that 'cancer seemed nonexistent.'[1] "In 1904, only one out of twenty-four Americans had cancer in their lifetime. Now the cancer rate is one out of two in men and one out of three in women."[2] But it is now clear to everyone in the western world that diseases of all kinds are rampant and treatment of disease has become a problem as well as a huge industry.

By the 1990s, one out of five Americans under the age of 17 already had a chronic disease; 22% of Americans suffered from allergies; 60% had defective vision; 50% had

---

1   Moss, Ralph. *The War on Cancer*. Townsend Letter for Doctors and Patients. Nov. 2002

2   Morrison-Kelley, Carol. MD, FACC. Kelley, William, D. DDS, MS. *Cancer Ignorance, Part I*. http://www.whale.to/cancer/kelley/ci.html

chronic digestive disorders; and 9 out of 10 suffered from clogged colons.[3]

The World Health Organization report of June 4, 2000 listed healthy life expectancies of people in nations around the world. Japan and Australia ranked numbers 1 and 2 respectively, Canada was 12th, and the United States of America was 24th. Dr. Christopher Murray stated:

> The position of the United States is one of the major surprises of the new rating system. Basically, you die earlier and spend more time disabled if you're an American rather than a member of most other advanced countries.[4]

On October 1st, 2012, CBS news reported that today's baby boomers are unhealthy and getting worse:

> Australian researchers from Adelaide's three universities have completed the first stage of a report on the generation born between the end of the Second World War and the mid-1960s. Obesity among baby boomers is more than double the rate of their parents at the same age, and the number of boomers with three or more chronic conditions was 700 percent greater than the previous generation.[5]

---

3   Robbins, Joel. DC, ND, MD. *College of Natural Health Extension Course*. 1995. Sec. I, p. 4.

4   http://home.earthlink.net/~acisney2/id30.html

5   Fearnow, Benjamin. Study: *Baby Boomers' Health Very Poor, Getting Worse*. CBSDC. October 1, 2012. http://washington.cbslocal.com/2012/10/01/study-baby-boomers-health-very-poor-getting-worse/

It's becoming increasingly evident that the symptoms developing are no longer just about old age. Young adults and children are becoming part of the statistics. This degenerative picture is by no means restricted to North America; it is being seen in other nations as well. The health situation is bad and getting worse, and will continue to get worse unless people wake up and inform themselves about why this is happening and begin to take healthy corrective action.

A book entitled *Death by Medicine,* written by Drs. Null, Dean, Feldman, and Rasio, first published in 2010 and based on an earlier study commissioned by the Nutrition Institute of America, concludes that: "the American medical system is the leading cause of death and injury in the United States."

I'll repeat that again. "The American medical system is the leading cause of death and injury in the United States."

The main reasons cited were: doctors' mistakes, adverse drug reactions, hospital infections, over-use of antibiotics, and unnecessary procedures, to name a few. These deaths are classed as iatrogenic deaths, which means "induced inadvertently by a physician or surgeon or by medical treatment or diagnostic procedures." In other words – mistakes!

A 2009 investigative report published in *The New Yorker* found that areas of the United States that use more conventional medicines and treatments tend to have worse health outcomes. In contrast, nearby areas with similar demographics but lesser use of medical procedures and drugs, tend to experience better health.

WE NEED TO CHANGE SOME THINGS FOR OURSELVES

It should be quite plain from that study that it might be wise to take a serious interest in controlling your own health. Self-care, based on sound natural knowledge, such as you are learning about here, puts you at the center of your health program decisions.

When you take control and make the necessary changes in your lifestyle to bring about detoxification and rebuilding of a healthier body, you move the odds of avoiding serious disease conditions as you grow older considerably in your favor. Wouldn't it be wonderful if you could reduce and even eliminate your dependence on drug medications just by changing the way you eat?

How did we get into this out of control disease situation?

Over the last few generations, as the medical system has changed, as more chemicals got introduced into our foods, as foods became processed for longer shelf life, and as we consumed more fast food, we became lulled into thinking that this is the way life was supposed to be, that science and commercial products were better than nature. Before we knew it, here we were in this disease-rampant society, bewildered, confused and wondering if we might be one of the lucky ones to avoid major disease. But the odds are stacked highly against us if we don't take responsibility for our personal health and change what we are doing.

How did we get this way, just accepting that others know better than we do, and that we should look to them for answers when we get sick? That we are not capable of making important decisions for ourselves? The quick answer is that we have been dumbed down – made to believe that we are not capable of running our own affairs. We have been taught not to think for ourselves. We have been conditioned from the time we were born. When we were children our parents gave us direction. When we went to school our teachers told us what to do and when to do it. At our places of worship the pastor, priest, rabbi, imam, or some other leader instructed us on what we should believe and how we should behave.

Later in our working life the boss set the rules – it was his or her way or the highway for us. We followed orders or we were out of a job. When we got sick people always told us to: "Go to the doctor. Doctor knows best". But does he or she always know what is best? Doctors emphasize pharmaceutical solutions. Now TV and other media tell us which things are good for us and what we should believe and what we should buy. We are subjected to a heavy and continual dose of brain-washing.

The end result of all this advice and direction from other people is usually confusion. We end up not knowing what or who to believe. When we are confused, we are open to being influenced and controlled.

The subconscious message here is that we need to look to others to make decisions for us, that we are not capable. But none of that is true. You are capable. You have a great mind of your own. You can check things out for the truth, including what you are reading here in this program. You need to know that the human body is wonderfully made. It doesn't make mistakes. We do. It has built-in wisdom on how to heal itself and stay healthy, but it can't do it without your help. You and the health of your body are a partnership. You have to work *with* it if you want real and lasting health.

THE BOTTOM LINE

In simple and brief terms, we have been purposely dumbed down, confused, deceived, lied to, manipulated, and directed by an industry for profit. We are the market. We are a crop to be harvested. If you don't believe that, just follow the money. There is far more money in treating sick people than there is in advising healthy people. As long as you stay committed to the sickness system, you are in someone else's power. There is a well-known quote that says, "When you know the truth, the truth will set you free." What you are learning here are some powerful and important truths about health and disease. You are being presented with knowledge, and knowledge is power – if you are prepared to use it.

We need to break out of our conditioning and see through the illusions that have been created for us. It is not what you think you know in life that's most important; it's the questions you ask. Ask the 'why' questions, the same as you did when you were an inquisitive little child. Little children are thirsty for knowledge and you should be too. Let me give you an example that I'll talk more about later. Do you read the labels on the food you buy and then ask yourself if all those ingredients are good for your body? Most people just grab it off the shelf, take it home, and then eat it. Be a questioner! Make decisions that are good for your body.

Who places more value on your life and the health of your body – you or your doctor? Now think about that. You do, of course. All you may have lacked is this realization of having been conditioned to believe in a certain way, and to look to someone else for answers. You have needed the knowledge to empower yourself to take control of your own health program.

As you work your way through this program you will understand that you CAN manage your own health. You start with little steps at the beginning. And then, when you go through a cold or flu as you do now, you will see these processes in a different light. It is encouraging and exciting to know that once you have given your body the healthy nutrition it needs, it will work to detoxify and re-heal itself.

MY PHILOSOPHY ON HEALTH

I want you to know that being healthy is not about giving up everything you like to eat or do. And it's not about hard exercise either. I believe that life is to be enjoyed. But we do have to find a balance. Having said that, in order to get our body on a healthy track, we first have to do some work to balance our internal chemistry and remove toxins that have built-up inside us over the years. I'll be explaining exactly how to do that in the rest of this program. Once that balance is achieved, we can be a little easier with our diet because after that we can monitor our chemistry and make adjustments as they are needed. It is all about being aware and conscious of what your body needs to keep you healthy and giving it the tools it needs to do its job.

As you move on through this program I want to tell you ahead of time that there is a lot of information here that you may not have heard about before. At first it might feel a little overwhelming, but don't let that discourage you. The solution is quite simple. As with all learning, repetition makes remembering easier. Just read the information several times until it becomes familiar and comfortable to you. In this way it will start to become part of you with a minimum of effort. I have done the work for you.

I wish you all the very best as you start this exciting venture into creating a new, healthier, and happier you. When you have poor health very little matters, but when you feel healthy and energetic, life is exciting. All things become possible again. And if you feel healthy now – great! This program can help you stay that way and move onto better levels of vibrant and lasting health.

In the second chapter I am going to talk about the wonderful human body and how it was designed to operate and serve us in health, and also how it can start to run into difficulties when we don't cooperate with it to supply what it needs to keep us healthy.

CHAPTER 2

YOUR WONDERFUL BODY
(and how we treat it)

In this chapter I am going to talk about:

- The wonderful human body and how it is designed to operate
- Why good digestion is so important
- How your body neutralizes acids within the digestive system
- The absolute need for regular elimination of wastes
- What your immune system needs to remain strong
- What proper chemical balance in your body is, and how this is related to oxygen and electrical energy
- Why your body's primary need is replenishment of electrical energy
- What your body's priorities for living are
- How your body heals
- Two important organs: the liver and the kidneys.

Caring for the human body can be compared to building a house. Once you have a building lot, two things are needed: construction materials and workers. In our bodies, the construction materials are found in the food we eat. To build a house we wouldn't use board scraps, burned pieces of plywood, wiring that has been soaked in acid or oil, or weak cement that has been mixed with one measure of cement to forty or fifty measures of sand or gravel. We would use quality materials to build a quality house that will be strong and serve us well for a very long time and also look good if it is maintained well. As we build the house, we would get rid of waste materials from the construction site and take them to the dump so the site is clean and the working environment is efficient.

To build strong bodies, we *also* need good nutrition from quality food, we need workers in the form of enzymes and probiotics from enough live food, and we need efficient elimination of waste materials from our body.

HOW THE HUMAN BODY OPERATES

The human body is a wonderful creation. We take it for granted that it is supposed to keep us healthy, regardless of what we eat or what our lifestyle practices are. As I discussed in the Introduction, we have been conditioned to think it is natural for our body to break down into various conditions of disease as we grow older. We don't like it and we are confused as to why it happens, but we reluctantly come to accept it as a part of aging. People say things such as "What can you expect at your age?" But that is misinformation and false programming. It is not the truth about the way the human body is capable of operating. The truth is at any age, if we give our body the tools it needs, we can expect to enjoy healthy longevity. We don't have to expect disease as we grow older.

As we begin to understand how it works, we realize what a perfectly designed and amazing body we have. If it is given the proper nutrition, exercise, and rest, and is supported by positive attitudes, and freedom from serious emotional stress, the human body is fully capable of staying healthy for 120 years or more, without serious aches, pains, or disease. It has innate intelligence, which means a built-in knowledge. It is designed to self-correct by instinct, automatically. All we have to do is work *with* it, not *against* it. Even in the face of all the wrongs we inflict on our body it still works hard to keep us healthy for as long as it can. It truly is a faithful servant. It is always trying to keep us alive for as long as possible, under the circumstances it has to deal with.

Our body's efficiency weakens only when we don't take care of its needs, or ignore the complaints it sends us in the form of symptoms. You see, these symptoms are a communication. Symptoms like a headache, indigestion, or high blood pressure, are our friends; they are not meant to be ignored. Our body sends us these symptoms to tell us that something is out of order. It needs our help to correct it, not for us simply to take a pill or have a procedure done to make the pain go away. Even when your body's efficiency is weakened it moves to a back-up plan, or I should say a fall-back plan, because it is going on the defence and retreating. At the same time it is still trying to keep the threat to your life away for as long as possible.

Examples of the body's back-up system

When your body's stored supply of the mineral sodium is exhausted, it draws on another mineral from the bones – calcium – to perform the function that sodium was supposed to. This process keeps us alive under these circumstances but with an eventual consequence, which in this case we call osteoporosis. Even cancer, that dreaded disease, is the result of an effort of the body to keep the person alive. If it didn't seal off certain toxins in a tumor for example, they would be free to circulate through the body bringing about death much faster as some cancers have their beginning ten to twenty years before the disease is usually diagnosed. Your body struggles in the face of deficiencies and hardships. It is very efficient. It doesn't make mistakes. All the while it hopes that you will wake up and supply the nutrition and lifestyle practices it needs to re-stock its toolbox of nutrients and help it to detoxify, so that it can reduce stress on its organs and have an opportunity to bring you back to health before it is too late.

Of course, the longer this ignoring process continues the less vitality your body has until finally it starts to break down and give in to disease. What else can we expect?

UNDERSTANDING DIGESTION

Digestion is *the* major starting point of health. All building materials for creating cells and tissues are broken down into molecular structures by digestive enzymes so your body can use them. Without these small building materials and workers, every cell, organ, and tissue in your body degenerates. Almost all people who are victims of degenerative diseases have problems with their digestion, and most of these can be traced back to a lack of digestive enzymes and weak stomach acid. If you suffer from digestive problems you cannot have optimum health. To improve your health you must work on improving your digestion.

Digestion starts in the mouth when food is chewed and mixed with saliva, which contains enzymes for digesting sugars. This is why it is very important to chew your food thoroughly. As food enters the stomach, hydrochloric acid and enzymes are secreted to combine with the enzymes already supplied in raw foods, or from supplemental digestive enzymes. Efficient digestion in the stomach is very important.

Partially digested food leaves the stomach and enters the small intestine for the final stage of digestion. The small intestine has an alkaline environment for this stage of digestion. Here, enzymes produced by the pancreas gland are secreted through the pancreatic duct into the small intestine. Pancreatic enzymes work only in an alkaline medium. Bile, secreted by the liver and stored in the gall bladder, is added to the mixture as needed to break down fat molecules into smaller particles. Digested food particles are absorbed in your small intestine and moved on to your liver. Using more enzymes, your liver converts the nutrients into usable energy and fuel for all cells of your body.

If we continue our intake of processed and toxic foods, drugs, and chemicals, our digestive systems fight a losing battle trying to keep us healthy. When we change to healthy lifestyle practices, our digestive systems can regain their strength. Symptoms of inefficient digestion include: indigestion, acid reflux, heartburn, bloating, gas that comes back up the esophagus, commonly called burping, and flatulence or bowel gas.

Everything we put into our mouths must be completely available and usable by the organs and cells of our bodies; otherwise the potential health benefits pass right through us. Our digestive systems must have their requirements met at every station along the way: the mouth, stomach, small intestine, and large intestine. It is the same as a production line for building cars. If the workers or correct materials are not available at each station along the way, the car cannot be built properly.

Health begins by eating foods your body can use *and* is able to properly digest and assimilate. When we are young we can usually get away with eating almost anything because our digestive systems are strong and healthy, but as we get older many people begin to develop problems with their digestion. We need to understand why this happens. It relates to a continual diet that is overly-acidic, causing a depletion of minerals from the body's reserves which are needed for efficient digestion. Overuse of prescription and over-the-counter drugs can also damage intestinal tract linings, which weakens the body's immune system and its ability to properly digest foods.

How your body neutralizes excess acid in your digestive system

This is extremely important and so few people ever even hear about it, let alone pay any attention to it. But when you understand this, you have one of the most important keys to stop yourself from sliding into what is called acidosis which, as I will explain later in this chapter, causes our body to have low levels of electricity and oxygen.

Under these conditions, disease develops and takes hold.

When a meal of mostly acidic foods, such as meat, potatoes, processed or fast food, along with coffee or maybe alcoholic beverages or sodas is eaten, the digestive system has some hard work ahead for itself trying to neutralize all the acids formed. It always tries to bring the system back to a near-neutral pH of 7, but with an overly-acidic diet this can be at great cost to its stores of alkaline minerals.

When your body is in a healthy state the fluid in and around the cells is neutral to slightly alkaline. The normal waste by-products from a diet of fruit and vegetables, plus wastes produced from exercise, are weak acids that your body easily eliminates through your lungs. However, acid by-products from the digestion of some other foods, especially animal proteins, are very strong. Your body needs to neutralize the acid minerals, such as nitrogen, sulphur, and phosphorus, from these foods with alkaline minerals, such as sodium, magnesium, potassium, and calcium from its own reserves. As discussed earlier, the more acidic our cellular chemistry is, the harder our bodies have to work to try to neutralize the acidity. This process is called buffering and your body uses alkaline minerals to do this.[6]

When strong acids are produced from digesting and metabolizing food, organic *sodium* is used first to bring intracellular fluid pH up to 6.1. Notice, I said *organic* sodium. This is obtained from living fruit and vegetables,

---

6   Paraphrased from: *Correlative Urinalysis*, by Morter, M. T., BS, MA, DC. B.E.S.T. Research Inc. 1987.

including sea vegetables, *not inorganic* sodium, such as from table salt which the body cannot use. I'll tell you more about this later.

After sodium has done its job, organic *potassium* reacts with the now weaker acids to bring the pH back to a near neutral 6.8. When your intake of acid-forming foods continues to be more than the intake of alkaline-forming foods, your alkaline reserves of sodium and potassium become depleted. Your body is then forced to move to its backup buffer system which requires the withdrawal of calcium from its bones. If your body is forced to continue this backup buffer process due to there not being enough alkaline foods in your diet, serious bone loss will result. According to Dr. Morter:

> Anyone who eats more than 47 grams of protein a day— no matter what the source of the protein—will eventually develop osteoporosis.[7]

Proteins cause strong acids to form in the body during digestion. Strong acids require alkaline minerals to neutralize them. High protein consumption continued over a prolonged period of time causes depletion of the first main buffering mineral, sodium. Once this mineral is not available, the body must draw on calcium reserves to neutralize acids. If you notice that many elderly people develop stooped shoulders and a rounding at the

---

7   Morter, M. T., BS, MA, DC. *Correlative Urinalysis*. B.E.S.T. Research Inc. 1987. p.51.

top of their backs, you can see the effects of their bodies withdrawing calcium from their spinal bones. Of course, it is also being withdrawn from all their bones as well, but this does not usually become evident until they fall and break one. The message here is that in life, everything in moderation and balance seems to work best. Work to keep your acid-alkaline levels balanced so that serious mineral depletion does not happen in your body.

You can see how important it is to pay attention to the amount of both alkaline- and acid-forming foods we eat on a regular basis. For normal health the ideal ratio is about 80% alkaline and 20% acid-forming foods. But if our body is in a serious acid condition, we may have to concentrate on almost all alkaline-forming foods – that is non-sweet fruits, vegetables, and alkaline drinks for some time, as well as taking an alkalizing supplement to replenish our store of alkaline minerals. Only in this way can the state of acidosis be corrected, and a reversal toward better health be accomplished.

Through the complete process of digestion, food works its way through the stomach, then into the small intestine, and finally moves into the colon for storage and absorption of water before being eliminated from the body as waste. This sequence of events is meant to operate with regular efficiency. If it does not, toxic wastes can be reabsorbed back into the body, causing auto-intoxication.

ELIMINATION OF WASTES
Let's discuss a subject that is natural for all of us but hardly anyone talks about – bowel movements! And because it

is not talked about very much, there is confusion or lack of knowledge over what is normal and how important it is to efficiently remove these wastes often. Having good, regular bowel movements is the first most important and continuing step in detoxification. Our bodies must be able to eliminate these toxic wastes from the colon that are created from food digestion and chemicals we eat with food, and from toxic air we breathe. If we do not have regular and efficient bowel movements, poisons that are held in the colon for too long are re-absorbed through the colon membranes and veins back into the body where they begin to affect our other tissues and organs.

The main avenue for the removal of wastes is by bowel movements through the colon. When the colon becomes burdened with too many wastes, it becomes clogged, which then starts to back-up and congest the liver. Then your body is forced to use other avenues such as your lungs and your kidneys to eliminate toxins. When it still has good energy the body uses mucus membranes and the skin as avenues of elimination as well. Colds, sinus problems, ear infections, measles, chicken pox, and eczema are examples of mucus and skin eliminations. As the body's vitality gets lower, it can no longer afford the expenditure of energy required for this alternate elimination anymore, so it is forced to store toxins in its tissues. As this process continues, toxins stored in the deeper tissues can eventually cause diseases such as arthritis, heart disease, senility, and cancer.

You should have two or three bowel movements each day. If you are a person who only has one or two bowel movements each week, you should be working to correct this as the first and highest priority because poisons are building up in your body – big time! In a later chapter on digestion and detoxification I will tell you about the various ways to do this. Stools should be well-formed, dark brown in color, contain no undigested food particles and be easy to pass. The whole elimination should take only a minute or two. When the number of movements is less than two or three times per day, a condition of stagnation exists. Wherever there is stagnant food matter, there is fermentation and rotting. That's what foul bathroom odour is all about. And where there is rotting, more toxins are formed.

When fecal matter sits in the colon for longer than normal, toxins are absorbed back into the body causing autointoxication, which is self-poisoning. Poisoning leads to disease. An example is that diverticula pockets – saclike hernias – in the colon, which may have been there for many years, can lead to colon cancer. From this progression we can understand the phrase used by many natural health practitioners that: "Disease begins in the colon." That is why it is so important to have regular and complete bowel movements. By keeping the colon free of stagnant wastes, we can turn the last phrase around to say: "Disease is prevented in the colon."

Good elimination depends on the many digestive processes that happen in the stomach and small intestine above the colon. It is also affected by the quality of food we eat, the digestive enzymes and probiotics present, how well food is chewed to break it down and mix it with saliva, our intake of enough water and fiber in our diet, and from the amount of moderate exercise we get.

Without regular and healthy bowel movements, a body cannot be truly healthy. We should observe our bowel movements regularly to be aware of what and how well we are digesting our food and eliminating wastes. This is an important part of being conscious and aware of your state of health.

THE IMMUNE SYSTEM

The immune system is a wonderfully balanced defence system in your body whose function is to defend against toxic invaders and to fight disease. It works to eliminate harmful substances that shouldn't be there such as drugs, pollens, insect venom, chemicals in foods, diseased cells, and anything that is unnatural to your body. It can deal with a wide range of agents that cause disease such as viruses, bacteria, fungi, and parasites. We are meant to obtain essential immunity factors from colostrum in our mother's milk during our first feedings just after we are born.

Our bodies have two kinds of immunity. Everyone is born with a built-in immunity – the ability to react to foreign substances. But our bodies also have learned immunity, which is the ability to adapt and remember. This explains why people do not get chickenpox or measles more than once.

As great as the immune system is, it can only work if it is cared for properly. This means getting healthy nutrition and enzymes, and having a clean colon and liver free of too many toxins. We also need to avoid those things that tend to depress immunity such as: some household cleaners, overuse of antibiotics and drugs, mercury in tooth fillings, pesticides, chemical additives in foods we eat, exposure to air pollutants, and too much stress.

Strong immunity is also dependent on your having a healthy supply of good bacteria, called probiotics, in your intestines. However, many of our common lifestyle practices work against a strong immune system. I will talk more about these in the next chapter when I discuss some of the main things we do that undermine our health.

The purpose of a fever

One of the most powerful weapons your body uses to overcome viruses is a fever. Some people think that a fever is bad, but fevers in the range of 102 or 103 degrees Fahrenheit (39°C) can be good – they are actually part of the body's natural defense against invading viruses. Viruses multiply very well at the normal body temperature of 98.6°F or 37°C. However, they are not able to live and multiply at temperatures above 101°F or 38.3°C. But, when we take medications such as aspirin or other anti-inflammatory drugs, which contain acetylsalicylic acid, to feel temporary relief, we interfere with this natural process. We may feel some temporary relief from pain or stuffiness, but these medications also lower the body's fever below 100°F or (37.8°C). At this body temperature the viruses are free to multiply unchallenged and spread throughout the body.

A young or relatively healthy body may be able to handle this interference, but the elderly and those with weak immune systems may develop a serious condition such as pneumonia, which can lead to death. There is research which states that the cause of millions of deaths from the 1918 flu epidemic was not the flu virus, but the widespread use of aspirin during this time.[8] A body trying to fight viruses at low temperatures is fighting a losing battle.

Why do some people develop diseases?

The human body has a tremendous built-in ability and corrective capability, but it has limits. If deficiencies are not corrected, and abuses are not stopped, sooner or later it will begin to break down and health disturbances will start to appear in some area of the body. The location is often related to genetic or inherited weaknesses passed on from our parents and grandparents. The disease conditions often appear because we tend to carry food and eating preferences similar to what we were raised with. Under stress, these areas tend to be the first to show signs of disease such as allergy, asthma, high blood pressure, heart disease, arthritis, diabetes, and emotional disorders. If you work with your body to supply what it needs, those inherited family health weaknesses do not need to develop at all. Your body will naturally strengthen itself in those areas.

You can be your body's greatest friend or its worst enemy. Your choices of food, rest, exercise, fresh air, sunshine, and attitudes have the greatest impacts on your health. We need to know *what* our bodies require to be healthy. We need to understand how our bodies function.

---

8   Starks, Karen M., *Salicylates and Pandemic Influenza Mortality, 1918–1919 Pharmacology, Pathology, and Historic Evidence*. 2009 http://bit.ly/Rm4xx2

CORRECT CHEMICAL BALANCE

The human body was designed to operate most efficiently in a certain chemical balance. Chemical balance and electrical energy in the body go hand in hand – imbalance in one, negatively affects the other. We call this chemical balance 'acid-alkaline' balance and it is most directly related to the kinds of food and beverages we consume. First, I will explain how we measure acid and alkaline.

Back in high school chemistry we learned that acid-alkaline strength is measured by pH. You could think of pH as standing for potential hydrogen ions, or it could stand for potential health because it is so critically important to health. The pH scale runs from 0 to 14. Zero is the most acidic and 14 the most alkaline, 7 is neutral. Balanced liquids have a neutral pH of 7. A small change in pH has a large effect in your body. This is because the pH scale for acid-alkaline is similar to the Richter scale for measuring the strength of earthquakes. Each one-point change in the scale results in a tenfold change in strength. For example, a pH change going from of 7.0 to 6.0 indicates an effective acid strength of ten, while an acid reading of pH 5.0 would be ten times as strong again, with a strength of one hundred – that is, (10 x 10). Similarly, as a fluid pH moves upward on the scale past 7.0, it increases the same way in alkaline strength.

The acid or alkaline strength in your body directly relates to levels of oxygen and electrical strength. The more acidic your body becomes, the less oxygen and electrons it has. As your body is able to move toward the neutral pH 7 or even slightly alkaline, the more oxygen and electrons it has, and the healthier you are. Everything in your body works well at this level. Let's consider why oxygen is so important.

Oxygen is the big key

Without oxygen we would all die within a few minutes. This most important nutrient for our body gives us a big clue to a secret of health. When the oxygen content in and around the cells of our bodies is high, symptoms of disease do not happen. In fact, Dr. Otto Warburg won the Nobel Prize in 1931 for discovering that cancer cells cannot grow when oxygen levels are normal. He stated in an article titled, *The Prime Cause and Prevention of Cancer* that: "the cause of cancer is no longer a mystery; we know it occurs whenever any cell is denied 60% of its oxygen requirements."[9]

Oxygen levels in our bodies are normal when cellular fluids are near to pH 7. As oxygen content and electricity decrease in your body, disease conditions increase. Viruses, parasites, and fungi love an oxygen-poor environment. As cellular pH becomes seriously acidic, around pH 5 or 4.5, oxygen levels are extremely low. It has been estimated that the cancer tissue in terminal cancer patients is approximately 1000 times more acidic than normal healthy tissue.[10] It is no wonder that cancer and the bad bugs take over under these conditions because oxygen levels are so low.

---

9   *Oxygen and Cancer.* http://www.cancerfightingstrategies.com/oxygen-and-cancer.html#sthash.ROTzfn6z.dpbs

10   *Low pH and Cancer.* http://myplace.frontier.com/~felipe2/id18.html

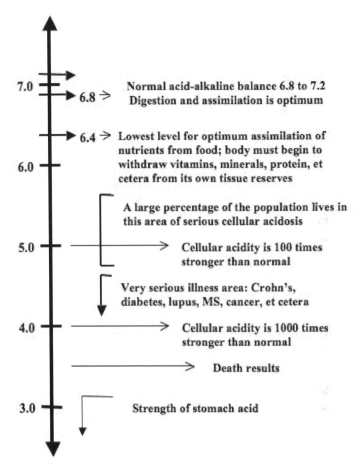

pH in Health and Disease
Diagram©RonGarner

Within the region of the diagram:

7.0
6.8 → Normal acid-alkaline balance 6.8 to 7.2
Digestion and assimilation is optimum

6.4 → Lowest level for optimum assimilation of
nutrients from food; body must begin to
withdraw vitamins, minerals, protein, et
cetera from its own tissue reserves

6.0

A large percentage of the population lives in
this area of serious cellular acidosis

5.0 Cellular acidity is 100 times
stronger than normal

Very serious illness area: Crohn's,
diabetes, lupus, MS, cancer, et cetera

4.0 Cellular acidity is 1000 times
stronger than normal

Death results

3.0 Strength of stomach acid

Without acid-alkaline balance we cannot achieve true health. It is that simple. The more acidic our body becomes, the less able it is to absorb minerals and other nutrients. The human body was designed to function best in a slightly alkaline state but it depends on us to supply its requirements of good food, electron replenishment, and positive attitudes. It always works for balance to produce good health. It never makes a mistake and always does what is necessary, given the circumstances it is dealing with.

In Chapter 7, I will tell you exactly how you can measure your body's acid-alkaline levels, right in your own home. With this simple method you can monitor your own health progress. This is an important step for you to be in control of your health program, and knowing when to make adjustments.

OUR ELECTRIC BODIES

Our bodies run on electricity. In fact, everything in the universe is an expression of energy. The whole purpose of supplying our body with food is so that it can be converted into electrical energy. The kind of food we eat combined with the efficiency of our digestive system forms the bodily chemical balance that must be maintained to create optimum health. The results of food digestion and assimilation directly relate to the amount of electrical energy or voltage our body has. Electrical energy in the body is directly related to acid-alkaline balance. This electrical energy is stored in your cells, each one with a positive and negative pole just like a little battery. So taken all together, you could think of your body as being a big battery like the kind we use in a flashlight.

We all know that flashlight batteries can lose their power and as this happens, the light becomes dimmer; the batteries have less energy. Our bodies are the same: if they are not recharged regularly, they lose their electrical life force. We become weaker, sicker, and less able to fight viruses and bad bacteria.

Our bodies have an electrical voltage that can be measured. As this voltage weakens, disease conditions start to appear. For example, chronic pain is a symptom of low voltage; we need electrons to heal. When we are not feeling well, we need electrons to get well. So the foods we eat are either electron *donors* – giving electrons to our body – or they are electron *stealers* – robbing electrons from our body; different foods are either making us stronger or making us weaker.

When voltage in our body drops, the cells produce less oxygen because they are becoming more acidic. See how closely these are related? As our body becomes more acidic, it produces less oxygen and has less electrical power. Our metabolism becomes weaker and bad bacteria start to multiply. As Dr. Jerry Tennant, the man who made an intensive study of the electrical aspect of the human body and discovered how it relates to our health, says: "The bugs" (bad bacteria) "are having lunch." So when you have low voltage, those bugs are having lunch on you! You need to get your acid-alkaline levels up so there will be more oxygen in the cells which in turn, will kill the parasitic bugs.

Recharging our bodies

There are two main sources from which we can recharge our bodies with electrons: unprocessed alkaline food and electrons from the earth.

Most fresh, raw fruits and vegetables are alkaline, with their living enzymes intact; they are electron donors. Alkaline fruits and vegetables can recharge the electrical body. Processed, packaged, canned, fast foods, and cooked foods are dead and acidic; their enzymes have been killed - they are electron stealers. If this is the only kind of food you eat all the time, your body's electron reserve is being drained quickly. Your ability to heal and fight disease is becoming weaker. It is like taking more money out of your bank account than you are putting in.

Also, food that has been denatured by the addition of chemicals and synthetic additives, and plants and animals that have been genetically modified, produce unnatural atoms that are not compatible with your body's natural requirements – the same as when a key won't fit a lock. So they also contribute to a lowering of your body's electrical efficiency and reserve.

Most of our fruit, grain, and vegetable foods are now grown in soils that have been stripped of minerals and treated with pesticides and chemical fertilizers. It is picked before it is ripe and has not gathered all its nutrients. Next, it is processed and had *all* its enzymes killed by being cooked in various ways. Commercial juices often have acid added to them and are pasteurized, which kills the enzymes, to give them longer shelf-life. Once again, we end up with food that, while it may contribute some temporary nutrition, is an electron stealer.

Everything done to food, such as processing and adding chemicals, changes its electrical nature. So, when it is broken down by our bodies for energy it is deficient in what our cells need for energy and tissue construction. This causes two things to happen. First, chemical toxins must be eliminated from our body, and if that's not possible the body stores them in its tissues. Second, our body is forced to rob the vitamins, minerals, proteins, and enzymes it needs from its own tissues, basically cannibalizing itself. Over time if nothing changes the body becomes weaker and disease starts to develop. Complete health returns only when your body's acid-alkaline and electrical balances are restored.

Let's go back to our house construction model for a moment. From the construction site analogy I talked about earlier, we can have all the best materials to build our house in a pile at the construction site, but if we have no workers to put the materials together they will just sit there and eventually rot. It's the same with our bodies. There are only two things that do 'construction work' in our bodies, and this is *very important* to understand: they are *enzymes,* and *bowel bacteria* or probiotics, the good-guy bacteria. Enzymes and probiotics are the active workers that put materials together and make things happen in your body.

Enzymes

Enzymes are living catalysts that activate all biochemical reactions in our bodies. Without enzymes you cannot see, you cannot hear, you cannot think, you cannot walk. In fact, without enzymes, body processes break down, organs die very quickly and death follows. So let me repeat: If you over-feed your body dead food, processed food, fast food, foods filled with preservatives and chemicals, you are using up your enzyme reserves in a hurry. It is like trying to drive your car with the gas gauge closing in on empty – sooner or later everything stops. I will explain more about getting enzymes into your diet in a later chapter when I talk about good foods for the body.

Probiotics – friendly bacteria

Probiotics work in the digestive tract, but mostly in the colon or large intestine. Pro-biotic simply means 'in favor of' or 'promoting' life. That's different from anti-biotic, which means 'against life.'

Probiotics are the good guys, sometimes called friendly bacteria, in your digestive tract system. Ideally, 'the good guys' – probiotics – should outnumber the 'bad guys' – bad bacteria – by a ratio of 85% to 15%.[11] Now with today's environment, diet, over-use of antibiotics, and antibiotics in meats, the ratio is far from this ideal in many people. That means the bad guys are winning the war and unless we fortify our army of good guys, we are creating disease in our bodies that could easily be avoided. For example, when someone has Candida – a yeast-like fungal infection – it's a sure sign that the bad guys are outnumbering the good guys in their digestive system. Every time you take antibiotics, they kill the good bacteria in your colon. So if you must take a course of antibiotics, make sure you also supplement with a good probiotic at the same time.

If enough friendly bacteria are not present in your bowel, your body can't make certain enzymes, vitamins, and natural antibiotics. Putrefaction, or rot and stagnation then happen in your colon and constipation results. *All disease symptoms*

---

11   The Answer to a Healthy Intestinal Tract. http://www.crohns.net/Miva/
     education/whatprobiotics.shtml

can be traced back to these problems in the colon, so you can see how important friendly bacteria are.

The main food sources of probiotics are plain yogurt, kefir, and fermented foods but fortunately, they also come in supplement form to help us keep the army of good guys in our digestive tract strong. I will tell you more about supplements in Chapter 8.

The bottom line on food is that we need enough unprocessed alkaline-forming food to keep our acid-alkaline levels balanced, our oxygen levels high, and our electrical energy up so that our immune systems will be strong. As to the liquids we should be drinking, there is a simple rule to keep in mind: the higher the pH reading, the more alkaline and oxygen-rich the fluid is. The lower the pH reading, the more acidic and oxygen-deprived the fluid is. From this rule you will see what huge electron and oxygen stealers all soda drinks are because they are very acidic, averaging between pH 3 and pH 4. This is over 1000 times more acidic than fluids at a neutral pH of 7. On the other hand, freshly-made fruit and vegetable juices and smoothies are alkaline; they help to restore healthy acid-alkaline balance in the body.

Electrons from the earth

The second way the body can replenish its electron reserves is from the earth. Be in physical contact with the earth as much as possible to help recharge your electrical system. As it happens, and it should be no surprise to us that nature has always been there to supply our needs, the earth is our most abundant source of healing electrons. All we have to do is make contact with it. In the book called *Earthing*, the authors say that the earth has an endless supply of negatively-charged free electrons.[12] When we are in contact with the earth by walking barefoot on it, or in contact with a grounding pad or grounding bed sheet that you can buy online for your home, we are taking in these healing electrons. They are like antioxidants that work to neutralize the harmful effects of pollution, radiation, smoke, and herbicides. No wonder that we feel good and energized after a vacation at the beach.

Another significant benefit of grounding is the ability of these electrons from the earth to neutralize the harmful electric and electronic pollution radiations in our homes when we are in contact with a grounding pad or sheet. When we are not grounded, every cell in our body is stressed by invisible electromagnetic fields generated by electrical wiring within the home, and by electrical devices such as wireless transmitters, smart meters, televisions, computers, cell phones and cordless phones.

Why this is so important is also because electrons from the earth are able to neutralize free radicals in our body. Free radicals are simply damaged molecules that are created from toxins in our body, and from electromagnetic radiations in our environment. Free radicals are always looking to be repaired and balanced again; they go though our body constantly breaking up stable molecules in a chain reaction. But of course this still leaves another single,

---

12   Ober, Clinton; Sinatra, Stephen, MD;, Zucker. Martin. *Earthing*. Basic Health Publications. Laguna Beach, CA. 92651. 2010. p. 64.

looking to be paired again. As it turns out, free radicals are at the basis of inflammation and disease. Unless enough electrons are available to your body to neutralize the free radicals, the inflammation process continues on in one form or another. Your body needs electrons to heal. So to make a major step in gaining electrons that will help your body reduce inflammation and fight disease, get grounded as much, and as often as you can!

Now that I have talked about your body's main requirements for digestion, regular elimination, chemical balance, and electricity, let's understand what its priorities are and how it works to heal various conditions that arise.

YOUR BODY'S PRIORITIES

Did you know that your body has built-in priorities for how it operates? Well it does, and they are quite simple and logical. As a faithful servant, your body's first priority is always *survival*. It will do whatever it can to keep you alive for another day – in spite of the terrible odds it may be facing. We have all heard of cases where people with a terminal illness were expected by medical authorities to die in a certain amount of time, but they lived on for a great deal longer. This is an example of how your body does not give up.

Your body always works first to survive and then second, to maintain or restore health. If it has energy and nutritional reserves left over at the end of the day, only then can your body direct its focus to healing. Did you get that? If you are eating electron-stealing food all the time and not getting enough rest and sleep, your body will eventually be short of healing energy. Without enough nutrition and rest, all your body can do is work to survive. It can't work to rebuild your health because it is just trying to hold steady and stay alive.

Your body works hard to maintain a functioning blood system, heart, liver, kidneys, and lungs because of their importance to your survival. However, its second priority of improving health becomes difficult in the context of a harmful and unhealthy lifestyle. Only when there are sufficient nutrients, good water, fresh air, rest, moderate exercise, proper elimination of wastes, etc., does your body have a surplus of energy which it can, and will, direct toward improving health.

How does your body heal?
Assuming that your body has been able to build up a reserve of nutrition and energy, it heals naturally and methodically in definite stages, but again, only *when* it has built-up enough nutrition and energy above and beyond basic living requirements. If our living requirements put too many demands on our body, then it is not able to build up a healing reserve.

Healing consists of a resting phase and a healing phase. During the resting phase our bodies store nutrients and energy in response to an improved diet and lifestyle; we notice that we are feeling better and we are encouraged by the changes we have made.

The healing phase consists of detoxification, destruction of diseased cells and rebuilding of cells. During this phase, the part of the body to be healed is brought into priority and some symptoms of earlier illnesses are reactivated. This is where we need understanding of this process and must be patient as our body goes through its re-building process. When you start your health program and begin to feel this happening, re-read the discussion on 'Turning the Disease Bus Around' in Chapter 4, so you will have the confidence to stay the course and hang in there as your body throws out the old and rebuilds the new.

When your body is ready, but not necessarily when it's convenient for you, it will start to do some active and intense detoxifying and healing. This is known as a healing crisis. The reactions may be mild or they may be severe. One should expect this and work toward it because the body's built-in desire is perfect health.

The most common detoxifying process utilized by the human body in preparation for healing is a cold. An episode of the flu can also be used. During a cold your body starts eliminating toxic wastes that have been held in storage. Toxins are transported to the mucus membranes where they are combined with mucus for elimination from your body. As it begins to make gains through detoxification, your body then turns its attention to breaking down and removing diseased cells, replacing them with healthy ones. This process takes a lot of energy and is why, that during a cold or flu, we feel we don't have much energy. Understand it is not that your body has less energy during this healing episode than before, but that it is directing its energy towards house-cleaning and rebuilding. When it has finished its detoxification objective for this time, it will return the energy back to your muscles again.

Now, going through the cold may feel the same as when you have been sick before, but the difference is that now that you have been giving your body good nutrition and rest, after this cleansing effort is over, your body is left a little stronger than before. Before you were eating well, these colds and flues were energy-depleting crises; they were *survival* crises. Your body was just trying to stay alive. Now that you have been eating well, they are what are called *healing crises*. You are on your road to more energy and better health.

Considering that your body's first priority is to survive, its first healing efforts will be directed to the parts of the body most vital for survival. For example, there could be a life-threatening disease such as cancer or a heart problem in process within your body. In its wisdom, your body will want to correct this first to ensure survival. And it may take several episodes of gathering energy and bringing on another healing crisis to bring your body out of danger in this area.

During this time, it is essential that you do not try to force your body by physical, herbal, drug or other stimulants, as to which part it must work on. Your body always knows which part is the most important to focus on. The fact that we may want to lose weight when our body's first concern may be to heal a disease condition in our pancreas, liver or kidney, must be considered. Looking thinner when a developing cancer might be threatening our life quickly loses its importance. Even though we may not be aware of the condition, and medical doctors may not be able to diagnose it in its early stages, our body knows. It has a built-in, innate intelligence. It will take the necessary corrective action as a matter of course without us even knowing about it, if we work with it.

Your body heals in cycles

It works on each priority area until it is no longer the highest priority, moving on to the next condition after that. Little by little, vitality is raised and overall health is improved. As conditions improve in each area, your body will cycle back again to work on areas that are partially healed to increase health levels further. In this way it gradually works toward complete health. We need to be patient with this process and realize how long it took for disease or poor health conditions to develop. They cannot be reversed or corrected in only one or two efforts by your body. As long as you cooperate with it, your body will continue to work on healing in its effort to restore health.

Before we finish this chapter, let's talk about two organs you should understand because they are so important to health.

The Liver

Your liver is the largest internal organ in your body and is located in the upper right side of your abdomen, mostly under the ribs. It is truly magnificent and definitely one of the master organs of your body because it performs hundreds of complex tasks every day to keep you healthy. Some of the main tasks it performs include:

- Converting food into nutritional substances for life and growth
- Producing bile, an alkaline fluid, to aid digestion by breaking down oil and fat molecules into smaller particles

- Manufacturing thousands of different types of enzymes
- Storing important nutrients such as glucose, vitamins, and minerals for use in your body
- Helping to filter many chemical substances, toxins, and waste products from the blood
- Manufacturing the basic starter hormones for the endocrine system.

The liver works well and efficiently as long as the diet is healthy, and *until* the colon cannot eliminate all its wastes. Then toxins begin to back up into the liver causing congestion and reducing efficiency. Chlorine and too much alcohol can also cause damage to this vital organ. As you can see, we need to have a lot of consideration for our livers because it is impossible to have a healthy body without a healthy liver.

The Kidneys

The kidneys are bean-shaped organs about four inches long, two inches wide, and one inch thick, located against the back wall of the abdomen at the lower rib cage portion. The human body usually has two kidneys. Their function is to keep the pH balance of blood in the body as constant as possible. Therefore its main task is blood filtration. After blood has circulated through the liver and heart it then enters the kidneys for purification. Your kidneys work to maintain proper pH balance in the blood by eliminating excess water, salts, and other elements in the form of urine. Your urine is a derivative of your blood and is not a toxic waste. It is a sterile and nutritious fluid. Depending on your body's needs at the time, most of the useful materials in urine are reabsorbed back into your blood stream. Minerals and other nutritional factors in excess of what your body needs are stored in your bladder before being expelled from your body through urination.

Kidneys that are stressed and under-functioning become that way due to an overstressed and congested liver. Therefore, the key to improving your kidney function is to work on improving the health of your liver. And the first step in improving the health of your liver is to have healthy bowel movements that keep the colon free of congested wastes.

Now that we have covered the main aspects of how the human body operates and what it needs to keep its electrical energy high and its internal chemistry balanced, in the next chapter I want to talk about the things we do that work against these body operations – the things that undermine our health. Becoming aware of the wrong things we are doing and why they are harmful is an important step in changing our lifestyle practices toward a healthier way of living. This is another part of being conscious about *your* health program.

CHAPTER 3

WHAT HAVE WE BEEN DOING WRONG?

In the first chapter I said there are two main reasons why we become unhealthy, either from lack of knowledge or laziness. Now the fact that you are reading this says that you are not lazy; you want to find out how to do it right.

In this chapter I am going to concentrate on the main things we do out of habit that are harmful to our body, without us realizing how they affect our health. I'll show you that if we do too many of them for too long, our health *definitely* will start to break down.

TAKING CARE OF OUR BODIES

We are supposed to take good care of our bodies. When one part of your body is stressed, the efficiency of your whole body becomes weaker. All parts are important. If one part suffers, your whole body suffers.

It is an odd quirk of human nature that we usually take better care of our cars and other machines, servicing them with proper fuel and parts. We wouldn't think of putting diesel fuel in a gasoline engine or dirty oil in the crankcase. Likewise, we try to take care of our household plants and gardens so they will produce good flowers, fruit, and vegetables. We wouldn't use salted water, soft drinks, or alcoholic beverages on the potted plants in our houses or feed them grease from cooking. If we want them to be healthy, we cultivate and nourish the soil. We know that they need clean water, air, sunshine, and agreeable temperatures.

Yet when it comes to our bodies we typically ignore common sense. We treat them as if they were super garbage digesters with stainless steel parts. We don't question whether the food we eat helps or harms our body. We dump greasy foods, sugar, salt, alcohol, harmful chemical food additives, drugs, and more into our stomachs. Some of us smoke, which is one of the worst things for health. We don't give our bodies enough rest. Some of us worry ourselves half to death on a regular basis. Yet we expect to be healthy. When we do become diseased, we think it is bad luck or that some germ or virus zapped us. But the germ or virus would not have gained a foothold in our body if our immune system, with its specialized cells to resist disease-producing organisms, had remained strong. Your body will be strong *if* you give it what it needs to be healthy, and *if* you keep it mostly free of toxic wastes.

In this program you are learning how to pay attention to your whole body, including the emotional part as well. So now let's turn to some of the main things many people do all the time that cause major stress to their bodies.

Personal responsibility

We take our health for granted. When we have health problems we have been taught to go to a doctor or take medication to make us feel better. However, judging by the disease rates today something is missing in the staying-healthy process. We are failing to take responsibility for our own health. If you are going to be responsible for any task you need to know what you are doing. Where your health is concerned, you need to become knowledgeable about the basics of what your body *needs* in order to be healthy.

HOW WE WEAKEN OUR DIGESTIVE SYSTEM

We can never have our best health without efficient digestion, and we cannot have efficient digestion without a good supply of digestive enzymes and sufficient stomach acid.

Our digestive systems become weakened when our body has been slowly starved of its nutritional needs for years on end; digestion gets weaker. It is not just what we *eat* that is important, it is what we are able to *digest*. Eating too many processed and dead foods that have no enzymes, eating wrong combinations of foods, toxic foods, stimulants, drugs, alcohol, and overeating, add to the load the digestive system has to cope with. This depletes your body's energy and stored reserves. Some substances, such as antibiotics, pain medication and genetically modified foods can cause Leaky Gut Syndrome, which seriously weakens our immune system. I will tell you more about this in Chapter 8.

The following are some lifestyle practices that cause stress to our systems:

1. Ignoring the acid-alkaline balance

We talked about acid-alkaline balance in the last chapter and how your body functions best with an internal chemistry of near-neutral pH. Now let's look at what we are doing that upsets this balance.

This may surprise you but the greatest causes of body acidity are stress and tension from negative emotions, such as anger and fear. Also detrimental are the acid-producing foods and beverages we consume. Ninety percent or more of the typical diet of most people is acidic. Considering this, the deck is stacked heavily toward disease.

An acid-based diet of overcooked foods, junk foods, sugar, dairy products, too much meat, soft drinks, alcohol, nicotine, and drugs of whatever kind, places an ever-increasing burden on the body. Dr. Joel Robbins, in one of his teaching lectures, cited this example of how acidifying some foods are: One meal of well-done steak with all the trimmings requires nine meals of fresh raw fruits and vegetables to balance out the acid introduced into the body from the meal.

Most liquids we drink are very acidic. A single 12-ounce glass of a cola-type soft drink upsets the acid-alkaline balance of the digestive system so much it requires 32 glasses of pure pH neutral water to bring it back into balance. That beloved cup of coffee requires 12 glasses of water to neutralize it. From the section in the last chapter on how your body neutralizes acids, just imagine how that draws down on your alkaline mineral reserves over time.

Beverage (glass or cup)	pH Value	Glasses of pH 7 water to neutralize
Coffee	5.2	12
Decaf coffee	5.0	12
Beer	4.2	18
Wine	3.6	20
Concentrated juice	3.2	24
Cola	2.5	32

Toxin storage in the body is also acidifying. Our body has to expend energy for digestion as well as elimination of toxins we take in with our food. If it is unable to eliminate the toxins because of insufficient nutrition and too much congestion in the organs, your body has no choice but to store them in its tissues where they will do the least harm for the time being. Your body hopes it will get the opportunity to eliminate stored toxins at a later date. But if you don't change your eating habits, your body never gets that chance. It keeps trying, by bringing on a cold for instance, to eliminate some toxins with mucus. But that only continues for as long as it still has energy to do it. When energy levels are too low, the toxins just build up in your system eventually bringing on more serious conditions.

An example of toxin storage can be seen in how the body deals with common table salt, sodium chloride. Refined salt, unlike natural sea salt, is unnatural and cannot be used by your body as a nutrient. Too much of it is toxic and harmful to your body. The body makes every attempt to eliminate it. But until it can be removed through the normal channels of elimination and through the skin with perspiration, it must be stored. In order to keep this toxic chemical from killing the cells your body holds extra water to dilute its concentration, which puts on extra weight. That is why we feel thirsty after a salty meal and experience some swelling of the tissues; our body is using extra water to dilute the salt.

As long as our diet remains mostly acidic, the alkaline mineral deficit problem will become worse and can lead to chronic disease. The more acidic our cells are, the poorer our health is. Eventually, when cells become too acidic, serious disease sets in and death follows.

2. Eating wrong combinations of foods

Very few people understand the principles of proper food combining, yet this is so basic to your digestion, the health of your body, and how energetic you feel. Animals in nature, feeding on natural raw foods, eat only one food at a time and never have digestive discomfort. This is the ideal way to eat and the healthiest for the body. But we have been conditioned to eat several different foods at the same meal. We can do this, as long as they are digestively compatible.

The principle of food combining is quite simple. In order to be properly digested, proteins require acid-splitting enzymes, while carbohydrates or starches require alkaline-splitting enzymes. When concentrated proteins and starches are eaten at the same meal – for example, meat and potatoes, or cheese sandwiches, or meat sandwiches, the acid and alkaline secretions tend to neutralize each other. When the digestive system is weak, this causes food to ferment and rot, producing toxic by-products. In the process, a person can experience indigestion, acid reflux, bloated feelings, gas, and nausea. As an example of this, try mixing baking soda and vinegar together in a glass with a little water and notice the bubbling and frothing; the gas produced is caused by an alkali mixing with an acid. They are counteracting each other.

Aside from the acid-alkaline digestion consideration, we should also become aware of the time that different foods take to digest. This is important because combining a fast-digesting food, such as sugar or fruit that has sugar in it, with a slower-digesting food, such as bread or meat, sets up fermentation in the stomachs of those who don't manufacture enough digestive enzymes and hydrochloric acid. This causes indigestion, which creates toxins that are hard on your body. For example, some people say they can't eat melons. The probability is high that they would have no difficulty digesting melons if they ate them alone, and not with or after other foods. Melons are sweet and complete the digestive process in the stomach very quickly – in five or ten minutes. But when combined with other foods which take much longer to digest, melons cause fermentation. The common practice of eating fruit or desserts containing sugar, with or after meals, is a classic 'no no' in proper food combining. It is just asking for trouble. However, most people do it all the time.

The following table gives a simplified general understanding of the guidelines to follow for proper food combinations:

FOODS THAT COMBINE WELL
Proteins + Salads (no starch)
Carbohydrates + All vegetables
Most dairy products + Salads (no starch)

FOODS THAT COMBINE POORLY
Concentrated Proteins + Carbohydrates
Fruit + Other foods

FOODS BEST EATEN ALONE
Melons
Most fruit (except apples, which will mix with
non-starchy salad vegetables)
Milk (if consumed at all)

The following are examples of approximate times for some foods, when eaten alone, to complete digestion in the stomach and pass into the small intestine. Although digestion times vary with the individual and according to the health of the stomach, these times can be used as general guidelines as to how much time to leave between meals to allow for complete digestion.

Melons – 10 to 20 minutes
(Watermelon, cantaloupe, et cetera)
Most fruit – 20 to 40 minutes
(Apples, oranges, pears, cherries, et cetera)
Sweet fruit – 30 to 60 minutes
(Bananas, fig, dates, dried fruit, et cetera)

Green and low starch vegetables – 1 to 1½ hours
Starchy vegetables – 1½ to 2 hours
(Potatoes, corn, carrots, et cetera)
Light starch (Grains, flours, et cetera) – 2 to 3 hours
Proteins (Vegetable–nuts, seeds) – 3 to 4 hours
Proteins (Animal–meat, fish) – 4 to 6 hours

If people ate foods in correct combinations and had efficient digestive systems, there would be no need for antacids. Food would be fully digested, broken-down, absorbed and metabolized by their bodies in an efficient manner without causing any discomfort. Waste products from digestion would be eliminated in well-formed stools that would not contain undigested fragments. People would be healthier, feel better and have more energy.

3. Overeating

We sometimes eat too much food at one time for our digestive systems to handle. Many people overload their plates, go for seconds and thirds, and eat until all the food is gone. They eat until they feel 'stuffed', or even until their stomachs hurt. So it shouldn't be surprising that many men and women have large bellies. Their stomachs have been stretched and stuffed repeatedly and their colons have become clogged with impacted wastes. They need to change their eating habits and work to detoxify their colons big time!

Overeating is stressful to your body. It is like flooding an engine with too much gasoline. When you eat too much food your stomach and your pancreas are not able to supply the quantity of enzymes and digestive juices required to properly digest it. The result is that food sits in your stomach longer than it should and does not digest completely. Toxins are produced. Your stomach, small intestine, and liver are over-burdened. Metabolic and toxic waste products are produced in quantities that your intestines may not be able to eliminate completely. When this happens, your body has no alternative but to contain the wastes in fat and pockets of toxins. These toxin pockets are what can develop into tumors and disease. The body is simply acting in a defensive manner to survive for as long as it can. If the body allowed these toxins to circulate freely in the blood stream and vital organs, we would die much sooner.

Richard Weindruch, suggests that a balanced, calorie-restricted diet should do wonders for the health and longevity of humans.[13] His comments are based on studies which showed that by restricting their food intake, the life spans of fish, insects, and rodents increased by 40% and more. In a study with monkeys, several measures of health, such as percentage of body fat, blood pressure, glucose, insulin, and triglyceride levels, were improved by caloric restriction. So the clear message here is that eating less is healthier.

A good objective for us to work toward is to leave the stomach 20% empty at each meal. This lightens the digestive load, greatly improves the absorption and assimilation of nutrients, and leaves more time and energy for our body

---

13   Weindruch, Richard. *Calorie Restriction and Aging*. Scientific American. 2006.

to properly eliminate waste products. By eating less food at meal times, and having healthy snacks between meals if we feel the need to, all systems of our body will work better. We will also have increased energy. We will feel lighter and livelier. All of this can contribute to better health and longer life.

4. Using stimulants

This is a big one and most of us use them far too often. I will touch on the highlights here. A stimulant is defined as: "anything which will cause a loss of stored energy in the body, while giving the body little or nothing in return."

Stimulants, such as coffee and nicotine, cause your body to speed up its metabolism because it views them as mostly toxic or undesirable and something which it should eliminate as quickly as possible. It does this primarily by producing *adrenaline*, which causes your liver to release stored glucose into the bloodstream. Cells then convert the glucose into energy. With this burst of energy and increased blood circulation your body works to eliminate the poisons that were taken in. Stimulants cause your body to go into an abnormal reaction. Basically, they 'rev-up' your body to run faster. They get you going and make you *feel* like you have *more* energy, but it is false energy. You are only feeling the energy lift because of the adrenaline. The stimulant itself didn't contain *nutritional energy* for your body.

Stimulants are harmful because they actually cost your body nutrients and energy in order to cope with the stress *caused* by them. The overuse of stimulants stresses your body by drawing on energy that could be used to improve your health; they deplete mineral reserves from tissues and bones. This leads to lower vitality and disease as we grow older. Many people get through the day by consuming stimulants in order to have energy and feel better. The most common are: caffeine, nicotine, sugar, table salt, and red meat. The first four of these contain *no nutrition* for the body.

The human body can only be stimulated for so long before it begins to tire and break down. For example, if you are riding a horse and want it to go faster, it will respond to the stimulation of a whip. But stimulating it repeatedly to keep it going at a fast pace will only work for so long. Eventually the horse's energy reserves deplete and it becomes exhausted. Repeatedly whipping a horse to make it run faster can kill it. It is the same with our bodies. They work as long and as efficiently as they can, attempting to respond to our needs. However, under the repeated whip of stimulation they too eventually become exhausted, break down, and die.

The good news is that if we stop introducing stimulants into our bodies, start eating alkaline, mineral-rich foods, get adequate rest and exercise, and remove negative attitudes, our bodies will replenish their reserves and move toward improved health and vitality.

Coffee drinkers force their bodies to run in high gear. Coffee has little or no food value. In order to rid itself of the caffeine your body produces adrenaline and draws glucose and minerals from its emergency reserve system. In this process your stomach temperature is raised, stomach acid increases, enzyme production is decreased, digestion becomes more difficult, heart rate is increased, blood vessels in the brain become narrower, lungs work harder, the nervous system is irritated, the adrenal glands, liver, and pancreas are stressed. Just one cup of coffee can increase your metabolism by 15%.[14] Too much caffeine stresses your body and causes it to overwork and wear out sooner.

Nicotine contains highly toxic irritants and poisons which are extremely acidifying and harmful to anybody. It overworks the adrenal glands and heart, constricts arteries, reduces circulation in all parts of a person's body and acts as a shock to the nervous system. One or two cigarettes per day can *block* the healing processes in a sick body. Nicotine is such a detriment to healing that one doctor I knew refused to work with patients who continued to smoke.

Common table salt, or sodium chloride, is salt that has been refined, processed, and depleted of its minerals. It is toxic and addictive. Refined salt is a chemical compound that contains no food value. It cannot be digested or assimilated. It accumulates in your body, is very acidifying, and causes disorders and diseases. It is harmful to your heart and has been linked to high blood pressure and hardening of the arteries. It places great stress on your kidneys and depletes calcium and potassium in your body, which can lead to osteoporosis and heart disease.

---

14   Bedwell, Sarah-Jane. RD. LDN. *Natural Ways to Speed Up Your Metabolism.* www.timigustafson.com/2011/natural-ways-to-speed-up-your-metabolism/

On the other hand, natural whole sea salt (not heated and refined sea salt, because there is a big difference), has many health benefits. It contains up to 84 minerals and trace minerals. Food should only be seasoned with whole sea salt *after* cooking, as heat harms the salt.

Sugar in all its forms is a stimulant so harmful to the body that it deserves a section of its own.

5. Eating too much sugar

> Science has now shown us, beyond any shadow of a doubt, that sugar in your food, in all its myriad of forms, is taking a devastating toll on your health.[15]

Sugar is something that most of us take for granted as being an accepted part of our diets, but what we don't realize is what a sneaky and deadly substance it can be. Consumed on a continual basis, refined sugar is truly a poison that undermines our health in so many ways. However, because it is addictive, we have grown to love the taste of it and even eat more of it as time goes along. Food manufacturers know this and that is why they add it, in all its various forms, to most of the processed foods we eat. Even discounting the amount of sugar that is in processed and fast foods we buy, our love affair with sugar has become so habit-forming that Americans and Britons now consume, on average, about

---

15   *Is Sugar A Sweet Old Friend That Is Secretly Plotting Your Demise?* The O'Brien Clinic. 2014.

22 teaspoons of *added* sugar to their diets *each day*.[16] So,[17] why is this so bad?

In her book *Suicide by Sugar*, Nancy Appleton lists 143 reasons why sugar is ruining your health.[18] I will not list them all here, but I will cover three main facts about sugar so you can understand how it is at the basis of so many conditions ranging from: tooth decay, mineral deficiencies, food allergies, alcoholism, wrinkled skin, premature aging, calcium malabsorption, gall and kidney stones, weakened eyesight, cataracts, bowel problems, arthritis, reduced learning capacity, fatigue, nervousness, depression, memory loss, hormone disruption, lung problems, heart disease, hypoglycaemia, diabetes, fatty liver, and obesity, to many kinds of cancer.

How can something as apparently simple as sugar be blamed for contributing to so many diseases? First, understand that sugar is not a food – it contributes nothing useful for the body to use as building materials. Refined sugar contains no nutrition. During its manufacture it becomes devitalized, demineralised, and robbed of any life-giving qualities it once had. Sugar robs mineral and energy reserves from your body while giving nothing in return. It is a simple carbohydrate that is digested and absorbed very quickly. The liver can convert small amounts of it to energy for immediate use by the body. However, sugar in

16 *Sugar Love: A Not So Sweet Story*. ngm.nationalgeographic.com/2013/08/ sugar/cohen-text

17 Boycott, Rosie. Mail Online. 2014. http://bit.ly/1qEnya7

18 Appleton, Nancy. PhD. *Suicide by Sugar*. 2012.

excess causes the liver to overload, which it then turns into fat that must be stored somewhere in the body – blood, tissues, and the liver itself. This can lead to non-alcoholic liver disease and insulin resistance. When this happens, insulin levels become elevated, which can lead to obesity, cardiovascular disease, and diabetes.[19]

Second, sugar causes inflammation in body cells. Inflammation is at the basis of most disease conditions. It is an immune system response to something ingested within the body that causes damage and must be healed. When inflammation becomes chronic, healthy areas of the body become damaged as well and can be the root cause of serious diseases such as cancer, heart disease, diabetes, asthma, osteoporosis, and Alzheimer's, to name a few.[20]

And third, the body's immune system is weakened as indicated in the previous paragraph. How serious is this weakening? It is estimated that one teaspoon of sugar weakens the immune system for three and one-half hours.[21] When you eat large amounts of sugar every day your immune system is always under stress and operating below its normal efficiency. The following chart[22] illustrates the effect that increasing amounts of sugar have on weakening immunity:

19 *Insulin Resistance and Prediabetes*. National Diabetes Information Clearinghouse. http://diabetes.niddk.nih.gov/dm/pubs/insulinresistance/

20 Drake, Victoria. J. PhD. *The Two Faces of Inflammation*. Linus Pauling Institute. http://lpi.oregonstate.edu/ss07/inflammation.html

21 *Sugar a Sweet Poison - Effects of Sugar on Your Health and Moods*. https://middlepath.com.au/qol/sugar_a-sweet-poison_effects-health-moods.php

22 Excerpted from: DeMaria, Robert. *DC. Dr. Bob's Guide to Stop ADHD in 18 Days*. Drugless Healthcare Solutions. 2005. p. 46.

Amount of Refined Sugar Consumed	Number of Bacteria a White Blood Cell CanProcess in ½ Hour	Decrease in Immunity
No sugar	14	0%
6 tsp = 8 oz of soft drink	10	25%
12 tsp = frosted brownie	5.5	60%
18 tsp = apple pie a la mode	2	85%
24 tsp = banana split	1	92%
[Uncontrolled Diabetic]	1	92%

(Note: A 12-ounce can of soda contains 9 tsp of sugar. An 8-ounce
serving of fruit-flavored yogurt contains almost as much)

Now as if sugar isn't bad enough, artificial sweeteners, which have been introduced into over 5000 food and drink products, are absolute poisons. During his 30 years of research on Alzheimer's disease, Dr. H. J. Roberts, author of *Aspartame Disease: An FDA Approved Epidemic,* states that artificial sweeteners containing aspartame, sold under various brand names such as NutraSweet, Splenda, Sucralose, and Equal, cause Alzheimer's, multiple sclerosis, lupus, chronic fatigue syndrome, fibromyalgia, vision problems, plus many other disease and dysfunction symptoms. Aspartame crosses the blood brain barrier and deteriorates the neurons of the brain. How does it do this? The methanol, which is wood alcohol, in aspartame is released when temperature exceeds 86°F (30°C). It then converts to formaldehyde and formic acid, which is a known carcinogen. When aspartame is consumed this always happens because normal body temperature is 98.6°F (37°C). Dr. Woody Monte, author of the book *While*

Science Sleeps: A Sweetener Kills, stated that: "aspartame is the most dangerous food additive on the market today."

So if you think it is healthier to substitute an artificial sweetener for sugar or to drink diet soft drinks, you should think again. Bringing on early dementia or an auto-immune disease is not something I want to take a chance of doing.

The message is very clear as stated in the quotation at the beginning of this discussion – over-consumption of sugar takes a devastating toll on your health. One of the most effective steps you can take to improve your health is to eliminate, as much as possible, all sugars and artificial sweeteners from your diet. Natural sweeteners such as honey and maple sugar can be used in small amounts. The same advice applies to most sweet fruits because they can contain high levels of glucose and fructose which can lead to increased hunger, the liver making excess fat, inflammation, and insulin resistance contributing to Type II diabetes.[23] Fruits to mostly avoid would be those containing more than half their natural sugars as fructose. These include figs, dates, watermelon, grapes, and most dried fruits, to name a few. Also avoid drinking pure fruit juices for the same reason. For example, it is better to eat apples and pears than to drink apple juice or pear juice, because whole fruits contain fiber that blocks surges in blood sugar. Check a fruit fructose-content chart online to determine the fruits that are safest to eat. In the remainder of this book I use the general term 'low-sweet' to refer to

23 Dolson, Laura. *Fructose: Sweet, But Dangerous*. http://lowcarbdiets.about. com/od/nutrition/a/fructosedangers.htm

these fruits.

Low-sweet fresh fruits generally include, from lowest to medium sugar content: Lemons, limes, cranberries, blackberries, raspberries, strawberries, peaches, nectarines, blueberries, melons, apricots, grapefruit, and some apples.

6. Too much red meat

The digestion of red meat produces strong acids even though it does contain nutrition. Animal proteins contain sulphur, nitrogen and phosphorus, which produce strong acids. That is why the body is stimulated to eliminate them. Therefore, it is wise to limit the quantity of red meat you eat. The advantage that eating some red meat has is that iron and vitamin B12 are readily available in this food, whereas they can be harder to get from vegetarian sources. Personally, I eat organic red meat once every two or three weeks.

Most cattle are given growth hormones and antibiotics to make them gain weight faster. When we eat meat containing hormones and antibiotics the residues are passed on to us, which can disrupt our endocrine system and add to our weight and health problems. We are also becoming antibiotic-resistant as a result of continually eating this meat.

According to the US Food and Drug Administration, antibiotic use on farms grew from about 18 million pounds in 1999 to nearly 30 million pounds in 2011.

Today 80 percent of the antibiotics used in the United States are fed to livestock. Theirs is a diet laced with low "subtherapeutic" doses of antibiotics, not to cure illness but to make the animals grow faster and survive cramped living conditions. The low doses kill many bacteria, but some develop mutations that make them immune to the same drugs that once destroyed them. ... As the use of antibiotics in farming and raising livestock has increased, new antibiotic resistant bacteria, or "superbugs" are emerging.[24]

The only way to avoid eating antibiotics and hormones in your meat is to buy *organic* meat, poultry, and dairy products. Also avoid farm-raised fish for similar reasons.

Now as if antibiotics and hormones in your meat are not bad enough, the meat industry has come up with another chemical that makes money for them but presents consumers with further problems. There is research showing that a drug called ractopamine is now being given to animals to make them more muscular and reduce their fat content. Ractopamine is also known to affect the human cardiovascular system and may cause food poisoning.[25] It is fed to a large percentage of pigs, cattle and turkeys. At least 160 countries, not including most of North America, have banned the use of ractopamine in food production.[26] The best way to avoid this chemical is to buy organically-produced meat.

---

24 Food and Environment Reporting Network. http://thefern.org/2013/05/whats-causing-the-rise-in-antibiotic-resistant-bacteria/

25 Embodys Wellness Spa's Blog *Ractopamine – Poison in our food?* http://bit.ly/1iUet8n

26 The Alternative Daily. *160 Countries Have Banned Dangerous Meat Additive Ractopamine: Why are We Still Eating It?* http://www.thealternativedaily.com/160-countries-banned-dangerous-meat-additive-ractopamine-still-eating/

7. Eating junk food

Junk food is called 'junk' for a reason; it does not provide good nutrition and often has a high content of trans-fats, sugar, salt, and calories, but is low in quality proteins, vitamins, and minerals. In the process of trying to digest and assimilate this substandard food the body actually loses nutrition from its stored reserves. Because of this, junk food contributes to disease conditions; it is missing part of the complete package of nutrients needed for health.

Although it is tasty, fast, and convenient, a diet high in junk food leads to vitamin, mineral, amino acid, and enzyme deficiencies. Junk foods are dead because they lack their live enzyme components; they have been refined, processed, overheated, and had chemical taste-enhancers added.

Foods usually considered to be junk foods include: candy, gum, salted snacks, fried fast food, and all carbonated soda drinks. Fast foods such as pizzas, hamburgers, hotdogs, tacos, and deep-fried foods may or may not be healthy, depending on their ingredients and how they are prepared. The more processed a food item, the more likely it is to be junk food.

The bottom line on junk food is that it is toxic and stressful to your body. If anybody wonders about this, check out the movie 'Super Size Me'. So here again, it comes down to your choice. You can eat food that nourishes your body, or you can eat food that puts toxins in your body which can lead to disease.

8. Too much cooked and processed food

Cooking and processing food kills the digestive enzymes in it. When most of the food we eat is cooked, our body must make its own digestive enzymes from its own body stores. Refining and processing food also destroys or distorts other natural nutrients. For example, refined white flour products such as bread, cookies, and pasta have been almost totally stripped of nutrients. Refined white flour contains only two or three nutrients compared to more than fifty in whole-wheat flour. Refined foods take more from your body than they give. When you eat them, they quickly convert to sugar, causing your body to take nutrients from itself to complete the digestion process. Over time, the depletion and deficiency of minerals such as calcium, magnesium, potassium, and phosphorus result. This leads to disease conditions.

Products that are labelled 'enriched' are no better. Actually, they are worse because most additives are toxic, forcing your body to use its energy and nutrients to eliminate them. In the refining process hundreds of nutrients are removed and then a few synthetic chemicals are added back. The food industry calls this enrichment. The products are not enriched; they are actually depleted and made more toxic by the synthetic additives. A study at the University of Texas in which rats were divided into groups and fed products made with whole wheat flour or enriched white refined flour, found that the rats continued to thrive on whole wheat, while those fed *enriched* white flour products either died or had stunted growth within ninety days.[27] The reason is because enrichment of this flour is from synthetic vitamins and minerals. Natural bodies don't function well on synthetics!

---

27 *White Flour is Killing You.* http://wholegrainalice.com/2011/09/white-flour-kills/

9. Too much protein

In the second chapter we talked about how eating too much protein causes acid conditions in body cells, which lowers oxygen production and voltage in cells. Scientific evidence from the medical community has found that the highest meat and dairy consuming nations in the world have the highest levels of illness and disease. Results of *The China Study*[28] by Dr. Colin Campbell,[29] conclude that chronic degenerative diseases occur at significantly higher rates where diets are richer in animal products. Excessive protein consumption causes increased metabolism, produces excess acids, and if continued over time, causes the pancreas to become overworked, enlarged and fatigued.

Once we have finished growing and have reached adulthood our body's need for protein drops. We need less protein percentage-wise than we did when we were babies and small children and were growing rapidly. In the last chapter I said that Dr. Morter found that anything more than 47 grams of protein per day, on average for adults, will result in a loss of calcium from the body, and if continued long enough *will result* in osteoporosis. However, the typical North American diet supplies 90 to 150 grams of protein per day. When we reduce our intake of animal proteins our requirement for vitamins and minerals decreases. This

---

28   *The China Study* examines the relationship between the consumption of animal products (including dairy) and chronic illnesses such as coronary heart disease, diabetes and cancers of the breast, prostrate and bowel.

29   T. Colin Campbell, PhD. Professor Emeritus of Nutritional Biochemistry at Cornell University in the United States, Dr. Campbell spent over 40 years researching, teaching and developing diets to optimize nutrition and health.

greatly reduces stress on our body and gives it more chance to heal.

10. Too many dairy products

The consumption of pasteurized dairy products can be harmful to your health. Besides having a protein content that is too high, most dairy products are pasteurized and they trigger mucus secretions in the body. Pasteurized milk contains no enzymes and is acid-forming. It is a myth that pasteurized milk is a good source of calcium. Unlike raw dairy products, pasteurized dairy products, in the process of being metabolized and eliminated, actually draw calcium *out of your bones*. This is caused by the acidic environment created in the body by the breakdown of milk protein.

Pasteurized milk contributes to many disease conditions such as: intestinal cramps, diarrhea, constipation, intestinal bleeding, skin conditions, bronchitis, ear infections, tooth decay, arthritis, and asthma.[30] I know of a young mother who was not able to digest milk products. One day, when her new son was five weeks old, she ate a piece of cheese pizza and an ice-cream cone. By the end of that week her son, who was breastfeeding, began bleeding with each bowel movement. When she went to the hospital she was told to stop breastfeeding and to put her baby on formula, and if the problem did not correct itself they would have to operate on the child to determine where the blood was coming from. She was not happy about doing this because she was very

---

30   Cassel, Ingri. *Does Milk Really Look Good On You?* http://www.all-creatures.org/cb/a-milklook.html

aware of the value mother's milk has in building a strong immune system for a baby. She did some research on this problem and discovered that pasteurized cow's milk can cause intestinal bleeding in individuals who are allergic to it. So this mother carefully avoided eating any dairy products and continued to breast-feed the child. In a few weeks the problem cleared completely and did not return. When a doctor told her that "it would be one chance in a million that her consumption of dairy products could be the cause of the bleeding," she replied: "Well, I guess I'm that one in a million," as she walked away.

As an illustration of how poor pasteurized dairy products are as food, consider what happens to newborn calves when they are fed pasteurized milk instead of raw, untreated milk. In 1940 an experiment was carried out by the West of Scotland Agricultural College in which two groups of newborn calves were fed – one with raw milk and the other with pasteurized milk.

In the raw milk group, all the animals finished the trial without mortality. In the pasteurized milk group, two died before they were thirty days old, and a third died on the ninety-second day, two days after the experiment finished. The remaining calves in the pasteurization group were in ill health at the end of the experiment, while all of the animals in the raw milk group were in excellent health.[31]

---

31   Schmidt, Michael. *A Tale of Two Calves*. Posted on December 10, 2010. http://www.realmilk.com/health/tale-of-two-calves/

And we feed these pasteurized products to our babies and children and expect them to be healthy and strong. More than that, we continue to eat and drink these same products as adults. Think about it. We are the only species that continues to drink milk after we have been weaned. And even then, we drink the milk of another species and pasteurize it to kill its life!

11. Soy and soy products

Boy, here is a big one! We have been sold a bill of goods by the soy industry that these foods are a healthy substitute for other foods. But the truth is exactly the reverse. If you have trouble believing this, do some of your own research online. You might start first by typing in 'soy and Price Pottenger Foundation' on your search engine. If you didn't know these facts before, you're in for a big surprise. Soy products, except the fermented ones such as tempeh, miso, and soy sauce, were not used as foods until their recent commercialization.

Contrary to popular belief, Japanese people don't live longer because they eat a lot of tofu. Traditionally, they have eaten only the fermented foods from soybeans as condiments with their meals.

Briefly, some of the negative properties of unfermented soybeans are that they contain:

- a clot-promoting substance that causes red blood cells to clump together
- substances that depress thyroid function
- enzyme inhibitors that block the action of other enzymes needed for protein digestion

- high levels of aluminum, which is toxic to the nervous system and the kidneys.

But perhaps my *biggest concern* about soy is that, due to the chemicals and high-heat processes used to make edible products from soybeans, such as tofu and soy milk, phyto-estrogens – which are plant-based estrogens – are produced. Non-fermented soy products are full of estrogens. These are not natural and they play havoc with a person's natural hormonal system. For example, as you read up on soy you will find the statement that 'babies on soy formula receive the estrogenic equivalent of at least 5 birth control pills per day.' I have first-hand knowledge of this fact because a girl in my family was fed soy formula as a baby and began to get her periods at nine years of age, due to the unnatural overload of estrogen.

12. Too many wheat products

Modern strains of commercial wheat have been re-engineered through cross-breeding and genetic manipulation to produce greater yields. However compared to older varieties, nutrient content is less and some gluten proteins are different and in significantly higher amounts. This newer kind of gluten, not formerly found in nature, is causing some people to develop gluten sensitivity or intolerance,[32] which can lead to various digestive tract problems. As explained by George Dvorsky, we do not have

---

32   Gunnars, Kris. *Modern Wheat – Old Diet Staple Turned Into Modern Health Nightmare.* February 2, 2014. http://authoritynutrition.com/modern-wheat-health-nightmare/

the enzymes in our digestive system to completely break this new gluten down. Consequently, it produces an immune response in the gut which increases intestinal permeability and inflammation that can lead to autoimmune diseases such as celiac disease, rheumatoid arthritis, and irritable bowel syndrome.[33] In these conditions gluten damages the lining of the small intestine to such an extent that adequate nutrients cannot be absorbed from food, which can lead to malnutrition.[34] This affects the health of the whole body with symptoms that can include bloating, pain, itchy skin, cramps, diarrhea, constipation, headaches, acid reflux, heartburn, and weight loss.

Gluten is found especially in wheat, but is also contained in other grains such as barley and rye. As alternatives, choose products made from other grains such as brown rice, or ancient wheat strains such as spelt and kamut. Among the best are millet and quinoa, which are actually on the alkaline side.

13. Drinking unhealthy water

Most tap water contains chlorine and sometimes fluoride as well, which are very toxic to your body. Chlorine kills friendly bacteria in the bowel and when it combines with some residues from digestion it forms cancer-causing compounds. Both chlorine and fluoride displace iodine in our systems which can lead to serious iodine deficiency and

---

33   Dvorsky, George. *Why You Should Probably Stop Eating Wheat.* December 14, 2012. http://bit.ly/1rjYPX3

34   *Wheat Intolerance: The Facts.* March 18, 2014. http://dailym.ai/1i63AmA

thyroid problems. Tap water can also contain pesticides and other chemicals. Also regarding fluoride, one should use only fluoride-free toothpaste.

Water from city systems should be passed through a good carbon filter unit to remove chlorine and other impurities before drinking it. A cheaper alternative can be a countertop jug or unit to filter out chlorine.

14. Overuse of prescription drugs

The conventional medical system mostly works with patients to manage disease symptoms with pharmaceutical drugs. When additional symptoms appear, more prescription medications are usually added. Once you are on two or more drug medications you often become a life-time customer of the pharmaceutical industry.

Drugs are unnatural chemicals which can alter the normal functioning of your body in some way. Your body has to use a great deal of energy and nutrients to neutralize and eliminate them. Antibiotics also kill friendly bacteria in your bowel that are needed for health. While drugs can take away symptoms such as pain, they do so by causing a greater stress or injury in another internal area of the body. Since your body only concentrates on the area of greatest threat and stress, the symptom for which the drug was taken is relieved and your body refocuses its attention to deal with the injury being caused by the introduced chemical irritant. However, the cause of the original pain or discomfort has not been removed or corrected. Only the symptom has been suppressed temporarily. It's like taking the battery out of your smoke alarm. The original problem is still smouldering away but waiting to break out at a later date. Not only that, but the body has the added stress of having to cope with the possible internal injury caused by the chemical drug. An example of this is that antibiotics and painkillers can damage the gut lining causing it to become leaky.

15. Getting too many vaccinations

This is a very contentious subject that is surrounded by a great deal of misinformation, advertising, and fear-promotion to the point of indoctrination and coercion. It is constantly pushed by the pharmaceutical and medical industries. However, research facts do not support the benefits that are claimed. If you doubt this, I strongly urge you to do a little research on your own. Check out the list of ingredients that are found in vaccines and decide for yourself whether you want them in your body. Research findings now available from many sources are indicating that vaccinations interfere with our body's immune system development and make us *more* susceptible to disease, not *less*.

There is a growing body of evidence suggesting that childhood diseases, most of which are harmless, are critical stages in the development of a strong, fully functioning immune system. Many babies are now vaccinated when they are just hours or days old. An immature immune system needs to develop naturally by fighting off illnesses that occur in childhood. Vaccines shield the body from exposure to minor illnesses but they may also be stunting its immune system and introducing other viruses and bacteria that the developing immune system cannot handle yet. Increasingly, vaccines are being linked to serious neurological disorders.

The question of taking vaccines is also an issue for adults. There is such a media blitz, especially toward the elderly, to have annual flu shots yet there is very little evidence that they are effective. In an article entitled *The Flu Vaccine Myth,* Croft Woodruff presents the case that flu vaccines may actually increase the risk of developing neurological pathologies. In this article he says,

> . . . according to Hugh Fudenberg, MD, . . . If an individual has had five flu shots between 1970 and 1980 (the years studied) her chances of getting Alzheimer's Disease is 10 times higher than if she had one, two or no shots. When asked why this was so, Fudenberg said it was due to the mercury and aluminum that is in every flu shot (and most childhood shots). The gradual mercury and aluminum build-up in the brain causes cognitive dysfunction. Is this why the number of those suffering from Alzheimer's is expected to quadruple?[35]

I am presenting this information for your consideration – to bring it to your attention so that you can make your own informed decision on the matter. I am neither recommending that you do or do not take vaccinations. That is your sole decision. However, I believe that you should be aware of the facts. As for myself, once I learned the facts I no longer take any vaccinations.

_____

35   Woodruff, Croft. *The Flu Vaccine Myth*. Alive Magazine. April 2000.

16. Not exercising regularly

Our bodies were meant to move regularly, not be inactive and sedentary. Many people today have office occupations or jobs driving vehicles that require them to be seated for long periods of time. This creates hardships for all body systems. Movement and exercise is one of the body's requirements for generating health.

Without regular exercise there is poor circulation of blood and insufficient movement of lymph fluids. Blood must be able to flow efficiently to carry oxygen and other nutrients to nourish cells and tissues. Exercise improves the removal of metabolic waste products and toxins from cells through the lymph system to the liver for filtration and elimination from the body. Exercise promotes muscle tone, generation of electricity and energy, and health of all body systems.

If you must spend many hours in a seated position, get up every hour or so and take a brief walk – even if it is to the bathroom or down the hallway. All body systems will benefit from this, including your brain, with the result of promoting better circulation and clearer thinking. Drivers who take the time to stop every hour or two to get out and walk for a few minutes feel better, have fewer back and bowel problems, and are more alert on the highway.

Exercise does not have to be strenuous. A half-hour walk each day is an excellent health habit. In addition, even five minutes or so of mild stretching, sit-ups, push-ups, knee-bends, and arm-curls with little weights will return rewarding benefits if done on a regular basis. I am an advocate of moderate exercise, especially for middle-aged and older people. Over-exercise can be harmful for sick or elderly people because it can be a drain on energy reserves. So, no matter what your present circumstances, try to incorporate even a small walking and exercise program into your health-building lifestyle.

17. Not getting enough rest and sleep

Healing can only happen when your body is resting or sleeping. Sleep is our time of 'battery recharging' when all conscious physical, mental, and emotional activity is suspended. This is when your body concentrates on cleansing, replenishing energy stores, and healing. Most of the energy we enjoy during the day was manufactured during the previous night's sleep. If you do not get a good night's rest, you cannot perform and feel at your best the next day. Enough sleep is also required for mental and emotional health. The amount of sleep required by a person depends on how toxic their body is and how much energy is being used up during waking hours. A detoxified body with a low-stress lifestyle needs less sleep to rest and rejuvenate.

In summary, if you don't get enough sleep for your body to recharge and rebuild itself, you cannot achieve optimum health.

18. Weakening our immune systems

In the last chapter I talked about the wonderful defence force we have inside our bodies. It is like an army equipped with natural killer cells. It is called our immune system. Its job is to neutralize and eliminate toxic substances that shouldn't be there. But if we don't take care of it, it will become weak and be unable to repel virus and bacterial invaders. It is just like the armies we have in our countries to keep us safe from foreign forces. If our country were to be invaded and attacked by foreign armies who had more and better weapons than we do, you know what the end result would be. It's the same with your body and that's why you need to keep your protective immune system strong and balanced.

However, without even realizing it there are many things that seriously weaken the ability of our immune systems to stay strong.

- Antibiotics, painkillers, and other drugs
- Chemicals and pesticides in our foods
- Radiation
- Chlorine and fluoride in drinking water and shower water
- Mercury in dental fillings.
- Vaccinations
- Too much alcohol
- Too much stress
- Too much sugar. One teaspoon of sugar will suppress your immune system for up to four hours.[36] Think what 8 teaspoons of sugar, which is the amount in most sodas, will do to your immune system and the ability of your white blood cells to overpower and destroy bacteria.

---

36 Colorado Center of Health and Nutrition. Side Effects of Sugar. http://www.fortcollinsnutrition.com/sideeffectsofsugar.html

When several of these factors are combined in your body – which is the case for most people, you can see how difficult it is for your immune system to be strong and keep you healthy. It is no wonder that our society is in a sad health state. As I have said before, your body is wonderfully made, but it is not a miracle worker. If you put enemies with stronger weapons inside your body, your immune system will weaken and the forces of disease will take over.

If you want to be healthy and stay that way, work to keep your immune system strong and balanced by avoiding those things that wear it down.

19. Living under continuously stressful conditions

This chapter is devoted to developing awareness of the major things many people do that place stress on their body organs. If these negative lifestyle practices are continued for too long they will lead to a breakdown of health and the emergence of various disease symptoms and conditions.

There is one other factor that is often overlooked and not understood when life seems so hectic and stressful that we feel exhausted. What I am talking about is adrenal fatigue, which can range from mild to severe, and to date this condition is rarely recognized by doctors in the conventional medical system.

We have two adrenal glands situated one on top of each kidney. The purpose of the adrenal glands is to help us cope with the various stresses in our lives, but they are responsible for much more. Hormones secreted by the adrenal glands influence all of the major physiological processes in the body including how carbohydrates, fats and proteins are utilized, stored and converted into energy. They regulate blood sugar, cardiovascular and gastrointestinal function. They also play a major role in controlling inflammation in the body and help to minimize allergic reactions.[37]

Our adrenal glands are meant to help us get through stressful events in our lives. We are aware that they temporarily produce adrenaline in response to events or substances the body perceives as threats to survival – the fight or flight response. Many years ago when life was simpler this response was typically a once in a while occurrence. However, our modern fast-paced life has changed that and many people are under regular and persistent strain which over-stresses the adrenal glands. When this is the case, the adrenal glands become tired and depleted, and so do we. In response to a very stressful or continuing situation the adrenal glands flood the body with the stress hormone cortisol. Normally, cortisol levels are higher in the morning to get us going and lower in the evening so we can wind down and get a good night's rest. But under the influence of chronic stress cortisol levels remain elevated, which wreaks havoc on the mind and body.[38]

Symptoms of adrenal fatigue can include: going to bed 'tired but wired', difficulty sleeping, waking in the night for extended periods of time, not feeling rested when you wake in the morning, feeling overwhelmed by life, memory problems, lack of sex drive, increased fat around

37 Wilson, James L. ND, DC, PhD. *Adrenal Fatigue, The 21st Century Stress Syndrome*. Smart Publications. 2001. pp. 3,4.

38 Bergland, Christopher. Cortisol: *Why "The Stress Hormone" is Public Enemy No. 1*. Psychology Today. http://bit.ly/1hl6ezR

the midsection, and unable to handle stressful situations without becoming emotionally and physically exhausted.

In addition to diet and lifestyle stressors listed in this chapter, our adrenal glands can become seriously traumatized by other factors such as: fear, death of a loved one, financial and legal issues, infections, serious surgical operations, verbal or physical abuse, unemployment, a difficult boss, and relationship stress.

People experiencing adrenal fatigue often resort to the use of caffeine, nicotine, cola drinks, alcohol, sugary foods, and other stimulants to get going in the morning and throughout the day, but this only compounds the problem and results in more serious health problems.

Once adrenal exhaustion has set in, it can take two years or more to be corrected. Strict attention needs to be given to: proper nutrition and other lifestyle factors such as you are being told about in *The Disease-Free Revolution*, getting extra sleep every night, and correcting or removing yourself from the serious emotional stressors in your life. When cortisol levels have become elevated, I have found the herbs Rhodiola[39] and Ashwagandha[40] to be very helpful in lowering them and helping my energy levels to improve.

If the discussion above seems to describe your own situation as a person who feels stressed and just can't seem

---

39 Gottfried, Sara. MD. *Cortisol Switcharoo: How the Main Stress Hormone Makes You Fat and Angry*. April 14, 2014. http://www.huffingtonpost.com/sara-gottfried-md/cortisol_b_1589670.html

40 Kiefer, Dale. *Ashwagandha Stress Reduction, Neural Protection, and a Lot More from an Ancient Herb*. Life Extension Magazine. June 2006. http://bit.ly/1ponqOL

to get your normal energy back, then I urge you to take the necessary steps to correct the diet, lifestyle, and situational stress factors that can lead to restoring the strength of your adrenal glands and improvement in your energy, health, and enjoyment of life. An excellent book to give you understanding of how to do that is: *Adrenal Fatigue, the 21st Century Stress Syndrome* by Dr. James Wilson.

20. Electromagnetic radiation exposure

This is a subject that people have heard about, but hardly anyone understands the dangers posed by it. Because electromagnetic fields and radiations are invisible, their harmful effect on living organisms, including humans, is being almost totally ignored. But it is so serious that a medical specialist is reported to have called the radiations emitted by mobile phones "the smoking gun of the 21st century."[41] He went on to say that "cordless phones and Wi-Fi work in the same way as a miniature microwave, emitting electromagnetic radiation."

Electromagnetic fields of varying frequencies are generated by the electrical wiring in our homes and offices, electrical appliances, computer screens, anti-theft devices. security systems, radio transmitters, television, radar, cellular telephones and antennas, cordless phones, microwave ovens, and Wi-Fi routers, to name the main offenders. The harmful effects of EMR are only just beginning to be recognized. Electromagnetic sensitivity has been associated with a wide

41   The Telegraph. May 30, 2013. *Are we ignoring the dangers of mobile phones?*
      www.bemri.org/news/mobile-phones.html

range of symptoms including insomnia, headaches, fatigue, poor concentration, irregular heartbeat, and dizziness.

The good news is that researchers are developing scalar energy devices to offer protection from EMR in the home. In addition, small personal units are available to provide protection from EMR when away from home. Three of my family members, including myself, have purchased one of these home devices[42] for our bedrooms and are very happy with the results we are experiencing in the form of deeper and uninterrupted sleep at night and, consequently, more energy during the day. Remember how important it is to get adequate and regenerative sleep, because this is when your body does most of its detoxification, healing, and manufacture of energy for the next day's activities.

HEAVY METALS - ANOTHER GROUP OF POISONS

The main heavy metals to be concerned about include mercury, nickel, lead, cadmium, and arsenic because they have all been implicated in human poisoning. Aluminum, although not a heavy metal, has also been linked to many diseases. In this discussion, I will talk briefly about aluminum and then mercury, because they are so prevalent in our lives.

If a criminal wanted to blow up or burn down a building but avoid suspicion by being well away from the area when it happened, he would plant a delayed action device. That's the way heavy metals, noxious chemicals, and pesticides work – very insidiously, like thieves in the night! They are very harmful to the human body. But they do their

---

42 www.freshandalive.com/

work in such a way that it is hard to connect the weakened immune system and developing diseases with the original or continuing exposure to the real culprit, because it takes so long for problems to develop.

Heavy metals can enter our bodies through food, water, air, and the skin – from industrial, pharmaceutical, agricultural, and dental sources. In our body systems, heavy metals compete with essential minerals such as calcium, magnesium, and zinc. This weakens our immune systems and causes imbalance and eventually, disease.

Aluminum

Aluminum is very common in our environment and has been linked to breast cancer, Parkinson's, and Alzheimer's disease. It is not needed by the body and therefore acts as an attacker – especially of the central nervous system.[43] This is why it is closely associated with mental impairment.

Aluminum accumulates in the kidneys, brain, lungs, liver and thyroid where it competes with calcium for absorption and can affect skeletal mineralization. In infants, this can slow growth.[44]

Aluminum's main sources in the body are from aluminum

---

43   Michalke B, Halbach S, Nischwitz V. JEM Spotlight: Metal speciation related to neurotoxicity in humans . J Environ Monit. 2009 May;11(5):939-54. doi: 10.1039/b817817h. Epub 2009 Mar 19. Review.

44   Global Healing Center. *Why I'm Concerned About the Dangers of Aluminum*. July 17, 2013. www.globalhealingcenter.com/natural-health/concerned-about-aluminum-dangers/#2

cookware and underarm anti-perspirants. It can also be found in aluminum foil, soda and beer cans, antacids, aspirin, vaccines, and in some brands of flour and baking powder. Once I found out about the harmful effects of aluminum, I removed these cookware and deodorant sources from our household. Stainless steel and glass, although more expensive to buy, are the safest cookware to use. Aluminum-free deodorants can be found in natural health stores. But here again, as with other products, read the labels to determine that they are toxin-free.

Mercury

Mercury has been labelled the most toxic non-radioactive metal known to humans. What is surprising about mercury is that its toxicity was well known in the 1700s, yet it is so present in our environment, industries, and medical uses today. What makes mercury so devastating to our health is its ability to travel to all parts of our body causing dysfunction, degeneration, and destruction of cells. Our immune systems weaken until we gradually slow down and then begin to see the rapid signs of aging in the mirror. Dental mercury-amalgams or so-called 'silver' amalgams and seafood, especially fish, are now recognized as the numbers one and two sources of mercury poisoning.

Silver amalgams used to fill cavities in teeth are mixtures of mercury, silver, copper, tin, and in some cases, zinc. All of these elements are toxic. But up to 50% of an amalgam's content is mercury. It is toxic in even small doses.

Dental amalgams are unstable compounds. They

corrode and the corrosion releases mercury into the body continuously. It is constantly being 'off gassed,' or released as mercury vapour in the mouth, and absorbed through the lungs and intestinal tract where it enters the blood stream. It settles mostly in the kidneys, liver, and brain. It is a time-released poison that is so slow and gradual there is little awareness of it happening. We rarely connect illness symptoms we experience with amalgams that were put into our teeth many years before. That is why this serious problem has been able to hide in plain sight for so long.

In a lecture I attended, Dr. Jerry Tennant, who I mentioned earlier, said that 70% of the patients coming to him for treatment are sick because of their teeth. The first thing he advises these patients to do is to have the metal removed from their teeth and have any root canal teeth they may have, extracted. These are so bad for health that he says many Integrative Medicine doctors in America now refuse to accept people as patients *unless* they have dental work done to correct these serious problems in their mouths. The reason is that any improvement they may be able to achieve with a patient's health will be quickly undone again by the poisons coming from their teeth. As long as their mouths are infected, trying to help them is a losing game.

Mercury is also found in some cosmetics, vaccines, and industrial products. Do your own questioning, research, and careful label-reading so that you can avoid taking mercury into your body.

Because mercury is so harmful to one's body, many people choose to have the mercury amalgams removed from their teeth. But, and I *emphasize this caution* – only have this done by a dentist who specializes in safe removal of mercury amalgams. This is because mercury released during high-speed drilling can be inhaled into the lungs and swallowed into the digestive system. Failure to take these precautions causes an immediate and serious poison overload in your body which can then cause you to feel sick, have less energy, and can lead to one or more of several serious conditions.

Root canals in teeth

The reason why root canal teeth are so unhealthy is because they have become a breeding ground for millions of harmful bacteria. When a root canal dental operation is performed on a tooth, the decayed root of a tooth is drilled out, including the entire nerve and blood supply that service that tooth. These are what give life to the tooth and when they are removed the tooth no longer has any natural circulation and immune system support; it is dead. Viewed under a microscope a tooth is very porous, like limestone; it is interlaced with a huge network of very small tunnels. When a root canal is performed, the tooth has lost its natural circulation of killer cells, so it now becomes a perfect and safe home for harmful bacteria to multiply unrestricted, and the poisons they produce leak out into the body. All root canals become infected[45] and in time, so does the bone around that tooth. This bone infection is

45 *97% of Terminal Cancer Patients Previously Had This Dental Procedure.* December 19, 2013. http://www.whydontyoutrythis.com/2013/12/97-percent-of-terminal-cancer-patients-previously-had-this-dental-procedure.html

called a cavitation, which is extremely difficult to correct. It is a serious and continual drain on the body's health.

Dr. Weston Price, the original researcher of health problems caused by root canal teeth, found that about 25% of the patients he treated, who had root-filled teeth, remained in good health provided they were not subjected to stressful problems such as an accident, influenza, or the death of a close family member. These individuals had excellent immune systems, excellent diets, and had parents and grandparents who were also healthy. If a patient was under stress however, or when their immune system was battling one or more degenerative illnesses, or if there was a history of chronic disease in the family, Dr. Price favoured avoiding treatment of infected teeth and recommended the removal of any which had root canal fillings.

Now the good news...
Dr. Hal Huggins, one of the authors of the book *Uninformed Consent: The Hidden Dangers in Dental Care,* reported that a number of so-called incurable diseases respond positively after all the offending dental materials have been removed from the mouth. Disease symptoms that have shown definite links to toxic metal poisoning are: fibromyalgia, epilepsy, leukemia, arthritis, diabetes, eye problems such as nearsightedness and astigmatism, high blood pressure, breast cancer, Parkinson's disease, allergies, blood cell abnormalities, lupus, Alzheimer's disease, multiple sclerosis, ringing in the ears, headaches, serum cholesterol levels, digestive problems, and memory difficulties.

In this chapter I have discussed many of the wrong

things most of us do in our society that place great stress on the ability of our bodies to continue producing energy and health for us. Once you are aware of these health facts, health is no longer rocket science but quite simple; it comes down to common sense. Do you want a healthy body? Or are you satisfied with being part of the usual slide into degenerative disease? It all comes down to what you want for yourself and how willing you are to adopt a healthy lifestyle.

In the next chapter I am going to talk about the important subject of removing congestion and toxins from your body – detoxification. It's mostly a what-to-do and how-to-do-it discussion. There are several aspects to this and I will try to tell you about the main considerations and ways detoxification can be done.

CHAPTER 4

TURNING THE DISEASE BUS AROUND

You may be surprised about some of the habits you have heard about so far that need to be changed. Nevertheless, you are gaining knowledge that you won't find on mainstream media or even from most health practitioners. You are gathering valuable information for your health-building toolbox. Creating good health starts with gaining knowledge and then following it up with action.

In the three previous chapters I talked about how the human body operates, what it *needs* to be able to produce health, and why it breaks down and develops disease conditions when its nutritional and lifestyle needs are not being met. Now we are moving into more of an action mode and what-to-do, as we start helping our body to lighten its toxic load. We are talking about detoxification and the healing stages your body goes through.

In this chapter I will address:

- The major negative things that we need to start correcting first as we begin a gradual process of changing over toward healthy lifestyle practices
- What we can expect as our body starts to gain enough

energy and nutrition to throw out the bad stuff in our bodies and then works to repair and renew itself. I call this phase of body work: "Turning the disease bus around"

- How long it can take to regain full and vibrant health
- Some of the best ways of helping your body to detoxify.

WHEN YOUR BODY STARTS SLOWING DOWN

In the second chapter you learned what proper chemical balance in the body is and how this is related to oxygen and electrical energy. Your body, with the exception of the stomach which secretes strong acids for digestion, needs to be as close to a neutral chemical pH of 7 for efficient health processes to take place. When it becomes too acidic your body starts to lose its ability to clean itself internally and most processes start to slow down. When the colon becomes clogged, congestion backs up into the liver, which causes it to start slowing down. All organs and glands are put under strain and are forced to operate with less efficiency. As this continues our bodies start to age and become factories for disease. So along with starting to eat better, the first thing we need to do is to help our bodies detoxify. Again, remember that you and your body are a team. It needs your help, just as much as you need it.

Reversing the slide into acidic body systems

The main factor in the weakening of our cellular system is the gradual acidification of body tissues. An acidic body is a body in which conditions of disease have already begun to take over. You might not notice it yet, but the conditions are there. The microbes and parasites that live in acidic, low-oxygen conditions are there doing their multiplying thing. They are already 'having lunch on you.'

All symptoms of illness and disease are related to too much acidity in the body.[46] Most disease problems can be avoided or reversed, but only by returning to a healthy acid-alkaline balance. The process starts with detoxifying your body to remove acid wastes. This eventually requires the elimination of all foods, drinks, harmful practices, negative attitudes, stresses, and environmental contaminants that have a damaging effect on the body. But we start with small steps first.

What are some of the things we should start giving up? And again, please realize that I am not suggesting you must do all these at once, unless of course you have a serious condition such as cancer that must be corrected. In this case you have no time to lose – all harmful foods and lifestyle practices should be eliminated quickly. Otherwise, take it slowly and 'pick your poisons' as the saying goes, for the first ones you are going to give up as you change over.

STIMULANTS
In the last chapter we talked about stimulants being substances that cause our bodies to increase metabolism to process them out. Stimulants trigger an abnormal speeding-up reaction in your body from adrenaline release as it works to remove toxins that the stimulants

46 Baroody, Theodore A. ND, MA, DC, PhD. *Alkalize of Die*. 2002. pp. 15, 185-187.

have introduced. In this process we can be fooled into thinking that the stimulant is giving us more energy, but the stimulant contains no energy. It only causes your body to use its own stored nutrients in attempts to eliminate the harmful substances. This results in depleted nutrient reserves and an early 'burnout.' As we saw in Chapter 3, the main food stimulants used in our society are caffeine, nicotine, alcohol, sugar, table salt, and too much red meat. They are toxic and very acid-producing.

When we stop putting stimulants into our bodies and start eating alkaline, mineral-rich foods, this immediately triggers a detoxification response by the body. It wants to move toward better health while it has the chance. But there is a temporary price to pay. Your body may have become dependent on stimulation from these foods for such a long time that it has become addicted to them. When we stop eating and drinking these foods the adrenaline rush is no longer there and consequently, the feelings of energy are immediately reduced. This is because it was actually false energy that did not come from nutrition. It came from a drug-like reaction, from a substance that caused the body to react in its effort to get rid of it. Eliminating stimulant toxins is a survival effort by your body; it can't use these substances for health and healing.

Consider the example of the person who drinks several cups of coffee throughout the day. When they go off coffee suddenly, by mid-morning of the next day they feel tired and irritable, and shortly after begin to experience a headache, usually across the forehead. The tiredness is due to a lack of energy stimulation from adrenaline release. The headache is from stored toxins entering the bloodstream for elimination and in the process, irritating nerves in the brain. As soon as the input of caffeine is discontinued, your body uses this opportunity to eliminate the poisons that had to be stored when the intake was continuous. In its wisdom, your body knows it must clean house because these poisons are threatening its long-term survival. After the main toxins have been eliminated, the uncomfortable detoxification symptoms will stop and energy will improve.

The bottom line on what we can expect when we discontinue the use of stimulants is some discomfort during the period of withdrawal. It may be preferable to eliminate the number and quantity of stimulants from our diet and lifestyle gradually. As an example, cut down the number of cups of coffee each day from say 5, to 4, to 3, etc. Take your time, but keep going down the list of stimulants you want to reduce and eliminate from your diet.

Over time, as stimulants are replaced with wholesome food, clean water, fresh air, moderate exercise, positive attitudes, and health-restoring supplements, your body will cleanse itself and start to produce increasing energy on its own. Organs become cleaner and more efficient, and then you can experience new feelings of vitality that are genuine and lasting.

The worst stimulant is smoking

If you are a smoker, you definitely should give it up as soon as you are able to do it. Remember from the last chapter that nicotine contains highly toxic irritants and poisons that are extremely acidifying and harmful to your body.

This should be near the top of your list to take out of your lifestyle. Two fresh approaches on how to do this include: a slow reduction of cigarettes and reprogramming your subconscious mind by repeatedly telling yourself, many times each day, that on a specific future date you will quit smoking and not need it anymore. One book by British author Allen Carr, *The Easy Way to Stop Smoking,* has apparently helped millions of smokers stop the habit without feeling anxious and deprived because it helps smokers discover the psychological reasons behind their dependency.

No matter what method is used, it is very important to stop this habit because a body will not recover health if one continues smoking.

Food Addictions

We all have our favorite foods. We can become addicted to certain foods for various payoffs, be they physical – we feel more energy; psychological or emotional – they make us feel better, calmer, and happier; or chemical – they satisfy a craving. When we have an addiction, the diseased or unhealthy part of our body is in control. It is fairly easy to understand addictions to caffeine, nicotine, alcohol, and drugs, but it is a little harder to consider foods such as bread, pasta, meat, and desserts as addictive. But they are addictive as well because of the payoffs just listed, in spite of the lack of nutrition they provide and the loss of energy they cause during detoxification efforts by the body.

The ultimate but not so obvious addiction that virtually all of us have is to cooked food. Addiction to cooked food is so ingrained and set in from thousands of years of custom, tradition, and practice that we accept it as normal. Newborn babies still have innate intelligence within them that finds cooked food repulsive. Babies usually try to spit out cooked and canned food preparations when they are first given solid food. After the mother's persistence and coaxing, they finally give in and accept it. It is not long before they *too* become addicted to sugar, salt, and cooked food. Humans are the only species that cooks its food. We need to use common sense regarding the amount of cooked food we eat, and we must work to achieve and maintain a healthy acid-alkaline balance.

While we are removing stimulants from our diet, we should begin trying to eat more raw fruits and vegetables and work slowly toward the 50/50 – raw to cooked food, or a little better.

WHAT WE CAN EXPECT AS WE BEGIN TO DETOXIFY AND EAT BETTER

No matter how old you are, one thing is obvious – it took many years of living the way you have been living to get to the levels of energy where you feel tired and maybe suffer from poorer health compared to years before when you were younger.

In the early part of life we don't go straight from good health to poor health; it usually happens in stages. Toxic accumulations from our lifestyle choices gradually reduce the ability of our body to be efficient. Over time its general immunity is weakened and it fights through each illness crisis by *trying to do* detoxification and repair. Each episode has a period of feeling sick (down) before returning to feeling better again (up). But as poisons continue to overload the system, each return to a healthy-feeling state (up) is achieved with a lower level of vitality left over. This is the movement toward degenerative disease. It is the slow, downward road to poor health.

Likewise, just as the downward road to ill health is not straight, the road back to energetic health is also traveled in stages. We go back to better health gradually with periods of detoxification and repair – first feeling much better (up), then having a cleaning-out and rebuilding period (down), then up, then slipping back. But each time, the reactions UP go farther than the reactions DOWN.[47] The body is gaining vitality and immunity as it cleans and rebuilds itself.

Complete healing takes time. Your body cannot restore everything at the same time. Some parts, some organs, some muscles are usually more deteriorated than others. We have to be prepared for some reactions and upsets on the road back to health. If we are doing everything right, these are simply healing corrections. The little periods of illness are natural times of thorough healing when strength and vitality are being rebuilt. Our bodies have to throw out the old and nasty before they can bring in the new life.

It can come as a shock to people after they have started to do all the right things and begun to feel much better, that there have to be downtimes of illness again. But our body corrects and builds toward health in stages. The road to normal vitality is not without its challenging times.

---

47   Irons, V. E. Dr. *Reactions*. Vol.IV, Number 5.2. Company Manual. pp. 3, 4.

Remember that true healing is not just the removal of symptoms; it is the complete and thorough reversal of the disease process. These episodes are called...

Healing reversals

When lifestyle practices that lead to disease are discontinued, your body starts by working to correct and remove disease conditions. This is called the 'reversal process.' There is no way that it can overcome or overlook the disease conditions that have become established within it without retracing them – that is, visiting them again to re-heal them properly. What went in must come out. A condition that built up must be broken down. Conditions that have been treated with drugs or antibiotics for instance, have been put on hold; a complete natural healing has not yet taken place. Only the symptoms have been removed. Disease conditions must be re-activated and reversed for damage to be undone. For example, when a person quits smoking they usually get a bad cold; lots of mucus comes up because the lungs are cleaning out.

The human body follows a clear pattern in the process of healing itself. The most *serious* and most *recent* disease conditions are given first attention. As progress is made on these, it works backwards in time so to speak, retracing and correcting other conditions in reverse order to when they appeared. Remember that all this is conditional on the body continuing to receive regular nutrition and rest, *over and above* what is required to carry on daily activities, so that it doesn't have to borrow from its own nutrient reserves to do healing. It always has to have energy and nutrition in its bank account before it can do some real corrective healing.

This is what healing is. There is no magic pill. Your body only builds from a firm foundation and does it step by step. The only way out of a problem is through it. And if you don't have a serious health problem now, these healing reversals will probably be fairly minor.

Each time your body has stored up enough nutrition and energy, and is prepared to do a healing reversal, it will bring on what is called a ...

Healing Crisis

A healing crisis is defined as: "an accelerated period of symptom reversal in a person who has grown strong enough to throw off accumulated toxic wastes from the past."

This is a turning point in the course of a disease, a period of necessary housecleaning as your body prepares to heal. It is the point you have been working towards, so don't be afraid of it. The most usual ones are a cold and flu. If a person has had a history of infections in some area of their body such as the lungs for example, then it will activate that condition to work on healing it naturally and properly without the interference of drugs, such as those I had to use for so many years. Other disease conditions are worked on in a similar fashion.

Your body can't go through this kind of healing and still be able to provide energy for everyday activities at the same time. Rest is needed. That is why we have less energy during a cold or flu. These are times of intense internal cleansing. Our *body* doesn't have less *energy*; it is just temporarily redirecting it for healing purposes. So when we are feeling tired during these times, it is good to remember that. When your body has finished its cleaning and repair for this time, it will return to normal. Energy and feelings of well-being will come back.

When we experience periods of illness and low energy, we might think that it is the same as when we were sick before. However, during a healing crisis there is one *very large difference*. This time, under the influence of a healthy lifestyle your body experiences symptoms related to a disease *healing* crisis, as opposed to a disease *survival* crisis. At the completion of each crisis it will have *gained* vitality, not lost it. Your body is getting *stronger*, not weaker.

The healthier we become, the less intense and less often the healing crises will be. This is logical, since the amount of toxins to be eliminated from the body is becoming less. The organs and tissues are getting stronger. And not every healing done by your body will slow you down like a cold or flu does. Sometimes you might just notice a little less energy or not feeling quite right for a short period of time. At these times your body may be working on some minor condition before returning to a feeling of renewed and energetic vitality.

As the physical body is being cleansed it can also bring emotional crises to the surface for correction. Old feelings of inferiority, sadness, depression, anger, and emotional conflicts *might* be experienced. These also need to be eliminated because in one way or another, they are connected to the development of a disease. I'll talk more about this in the next chapter on attitudes and beliefs. We need to be patient and work through these periods of emotional cleansing as well. Our body is working to return us to a complete, 'holistic' health of body, mind, and spirit.

Sometimes in the process of correcting a major problem a healing crisis can feel severe and be a bit scary. This is when you need to thoroughly review this process to understand how it works and what is going on. If it is *too* scary you may want to consult with your doctor about the advisability of resorting to the temporary use of some medication at this time. This will stop the natural healing process if it is necessary to restore your peace of mind. As long as you continue with your program of healthy nutrition and detoxification, when your body has built up its energy stores again it will make another attempt to heal this area at a later time.

How long do healing crises usually last?

A healing crisis usually lasts three or seven days. However, if there is enough healing energy available your body, it may run two or three healing crises one after the other. I had a healing crisis that lasted three weeks. It started with a cold and then advanced to a serious infection with a lot of congestion in my lungs. I was very tired and stayed in bed most of this time to rest. In the past I would have used antibiotics, but this time I let my body do the healing it was ready to do. After it was over, the serious lung infections I had regularly experienced were a thing of the past. This was a major problem that had to be corrected. And it *was* corrected because I had done enough detoxification and my body had built up enough energy from better nutrition.

My immune system was now strong enough for my body to carry out the complete healing correction. However, each person's immune system is different and you need to be confident that your immune system is strong enough to handle the healing crisis you are going through.

When your body brings on a healing crisis you should try not to interfere with this process by taking drugs to ease pain or discomfort. If this is done it will slow-down, and can even stop the natural corrective process. Likewise, it is not wise to stimulate your body to cleanse or focus healing on a part that *it* has not selected as a priority. If we do interfere, our body is forced to spend energy and nutrition dealing with the drug or stimulant. It has to change priority. Remember that your body uses its built-in intelligence to heal on a priority basis that is best for healing and survival. We need to work *with* our body, not *against* it. Let *your body* dictate what and when things will be worked on. It knows best, because...

Your body will start healing when it is ready

When your intake of healthy food is greater than your intake of unhealthy food the balance is tipped in favor of your body. It is able to divert some of its efforts away from survival toward healing and it will begin to detoxify. Toxins are moved from areas of cellular storage to the bloodstream for transport to the liver where they are separated from other blood components. From here they are sent onto the colon for elimination. During this process circulating blood passes though the body, including the brain. Toxins in the blood at that time can irritate sensitive nerves in the brain, causing a headache. In my personal case, when I know that my diet and lifestyle are good, the classic sign my body sends me, which indicates that it is detoxifying, is a mild to medium headache across my forehead. During these times I never use pain-killers. This kind of headache, although a bit unpleasant, is always tolerable and will pass when the detoxification cycle is finished. We can help our body to detoxify during these times by increasing our intake of healthy water, and getting extra rest.

Cooperating with our healing

During a serious healing crisis we should rest to save energy and eat quite lightly, if at all. All animals fast and rest quietly when they are not feeling well. This is the quickest and most efficient way to heal. Your body does not need food for energy at this time because it has already stored the energy required for the healing it wants to do. If it needed the energy from food it would not have begun the healing crisis in the first place. Continuing to eat regular meals during the healing crisis requires a lot of energy for digestion. Your body is then sidetracked from healing activities. It also interferes with the detoxification and elimination processes. Drinking good water and diluted freshly-made organic low-sweet fruit and vegetable juices is best, or eating a little broth made from an assortment of vegetables. In this way, your body is supplied with vitamins and minerals in non-solid form, which it can use easily without spending extra energy on digestion. Juiced foods require very little digestion.[48]

When nausea is present, it is the result of a concentration of toxins in the intestine. This can happen due to overeating, or eating overly toxic, or spoiled food. When there is a toxic overload being eliminated from your body, your liver, which normally processes waste products, may be forced to dump toxins directly into the intestines where they cause irritation and nausea. When this happens the last thing your body needs is more food. It may bring on nausea in an attempt to eliminate the toxins through vomiting and maybe diarrhea, or at least to signal that it wants you to fast – stop eating until it has re-established its digestive balance again.

To work with your body during a healing crisis you should drink healthful liquids, sleep and rest as much as possible, and stay warm. The whole intent is to conserve energy so that it can be directed to healing. You see, your body has only one pool of energy, and if you insist on forcing yourself to work, or exercise, or stay up late at night, your body cannot use that energy to heal you. In this sense, health is all about energy and where your body is able to use it. You can work with your body to heal and become stronger, or you can go against your body and continue to grind it down over time.

Also, as this is a time of increased dumping of toxic wastes, and if a headache is present, it is helpful to clear the bowel with a warm water enema once or twice each

---

48   Robbins, Joel. MD. *The Benefits of Juicing*. www.lchaimhealth.com/article9. html

day, or to have a colonic irrigation from a colon therapist. This helps with the elimination of toxins so they are not absorbed back into circulation around your body again.

If for some reason it becomes necessary to stop a healing crisis, this can usually be done by eating cooked vegetables, grains, meats, potatoes, or by drinking coffee. This will stop the detoxification process.

How long back to health?

This is always a question everyone is interested in. How long does it take for the human body to heal itself once we have started to eat properly and have adopted healthy lifestyle practices? The answer to this question varies for each person. Dr. Robbins, under whom I first studied, teaches that as a general rule it takes one year for every seven years you did it wrong. Dr. Kelly, who was an early successful alternative cancer treatment doctor, said that it takes 2 to 4 years to do 80% of the repair and rebuilding in the body, and it takes 4 to 7 years to do it completely. Healing is a gradual process, the same as most disease development is a gradual process. But don't become discouraged. Let's understand why it can take this long and how the time can be shortened.

The actual time required depends on how sick a body is in the first place and on how willing the person is to give their body what it needs to heal itself. It also depends on the disease present, how much vitality and digestive strength their body has, the person's attitudes, the environment the person lives and works in, how much stress is in their life, how quickly the person changes to a healthy diet, what supplements are added to the diet, and on their other lifestyle practices.

Disease conditions are developing in our body for a long time before symptoms even show up. Therefore, the body needs to go back in time to reverse and heal them. Serious problems take a long time to develop and are deeply seated. They cannot be corrected and replaced with totally healthy tissue in a short time. There is no magic bullet or quick fix that instantly heals anything. Healing naturally takes time, but it is methodical and thorough.

The sooner and more completely a healthy lifestyle is adopted, the sooner our return to health will be. For example, consuming fresh raw vegetable juices daily, with small amounts of juices made from low-sweet fruit for added flavour if desired, can achieve in one month what might normally take six months with a healthy diet of solid food to achieve. Restoring digestive enzymes, friendly intestinal bacteria, and consuming complete foods that contain alkaline minerals can shorten recovery time considerably. Again, it comes down to logical common sense.

Ninety-eight percent of the human body can be totally regenerated in one year.[49] So the answer to the question: "How long to health?" is that it depends on the age, present health, attitudes and beliefs, determination, circumstances, and capability of each individual. It also depends on our willingness to change our lifestyles to eat properly, detoxify, and spend the money required to restore enzymes, nutrients, and healthy pH balance to our body. It can take a year or two, or it can take ten.

---

49   Kestenbaum, David. *Atomic Tune-Up: How the Body Rejuvenates Itself.* July 14, 2007. www.npr.org/templates/story/story.php?storyId=11893583

For the average middle-aged person who undertakes a serious lifestyle change and does all the helpful things, it is reasonable to expect some positive changes in a matter of weeks or months. Significant changes can be expected in one to two years and a return to full health in as little as two to five years.

DETOXIFICATION

Detoxification is simply a process of helping the body to rid itself of stored wastes, congestion, and toxins that have been taken in from our foods and environment. It is not a one-time thing – it is a lifestyle process. After a while it will become just a routine part of your life.

When your body's needs are being supplied on a continual basis it detoxifies naturally as a matter of course. However, when there is a build-up of toxins from years of depriving your body of what it needs, and from abusing it with toxic foods, drinks, chemicals, drugs, smoke, and other stressors, it needs help to clean out and reverse disease conditions.

During the detoxification process we can focus mainly on removing toxins from our colon and liver. Once these organs have become less congested, other organs begin to release their congestion as well. So let's focus here on the benefits of detoxifying the colon, and then I'll talk briefly about the liver.

Benefits of Detoxification

The benefits of effective and regular detoxification are improved health, and that's what we want. When hard fecal matter, which is a mucus plaque that has built up on the walls of the colon over years is removed, our body begins to function more efficiently. Poisons and toxins are removed more quickly and good nutrients from foods are more easily absorbed as the cellular pH moves toward alkaline again. Digestion is improved. Immune function is better. The hormonal system works more harmoniously. The lymphatic system, which can be called the second sewer system of our body, becomes more fluid for effective drainage and elimination of cellular debris. We start to notice a difference because we have more energy and feel better.

Colon cleansing

As long as the colon is toxic, the liver and other organs will remain congested. Once we clear out the pollution at the 'bottom end,' the pressure is relieved, and the rest of our body is able to start dumping its toxins. This will be an ongoing program for quite some time because it can take several years to fully clean a body that has been toxic all its life. A diet that includes enough fiber from raw fruits and vegetables is the best and most natural colon cleanser and should always be the first priority for colon health. There are also several herbal colon-cleansing and rejuvenating products available in health food stores, as well as advertised on the Internet. I use a product called Herb Cocktail. While cleansing the colon of impacted debris we should be increasing our friendly flora probiotics to restore healthy bacteria in the digestive tract and colon.

Colon therapy can be a shortcut to health

Detoxification of body organs and tissues will normally

happen under a program of raw fruits, vegetables, good
water, and exercise. However, to really speed the process
up and assist your body toward health and reverse aging,
nothing is more immediately effective than thorough colon
therapy. This means the use of enemas or colonics, which I
will explain in the next sections.

Enemas

Although they reach only the lower portion of the colon,
enemas can be a great help. There are two main kinds
of enemas: clear water; and diluted coffee, the caffeine
kind, not decaffeinated, enemas, both taken at near to
body temperature. The great advantage of enemas is that
they can be done by yourself in the privacy of your own
home. Gentle massaging of your abdominal area during
the enema is also helpful. Detailed instructions on how to
use an enema can be found in Appendix 9. Enema kits are
usually available at most drug stores.

Clear water enemas are used to quickly flush the lower
section of the colon.   Coffee enemas are meant to be
retained in the colon for ten or fifteen minutes while some
of the caffeine is absorbed into the liver through connecting
veins for detoxification benefits.

Clear water enemas

Clear water is introduced into the colon and expelled again
fairly quickly, which provides a dilution and flushing of fecal matter in the lower portion of the colon. This kind of
enema can be repeated two or three times as necessary to
provide relief. During times of constipation or illness they

can be quite helpful because toxins in the colon are flushed out before they have a chance to be absorbed back into your body again.

Coffee enemas on the other hand, are usually held in the colon for about fifteen minutes before being expelled. These are called coffee retention enemas. A cup of caffeinated coffee is diluted by adding another two or three cups of filtered or distilled water and poured into an enema bag.

Coffee has been known for thousands of years as a potent liver remedy and has been given to the elderly and to those who were ill with liver problems. This is important for us today because almost everyone has a toxic liver. These enemas work effectively because the caffeine in coffee is drawn from the colon through veins into the liver where it is held for a few minutes. You will recall from an earlier chapter that the human body views caffeine as a toxin that it wants to get rid of. So along with its urge to eliminate caffeine, the liver is also stimulated to send other toxins out along with it. Many alternative cancer doctors and clinics recommend the use of two or three coffee enemas each day for their patients. However, for a normal detoxification program, a daily or every other day coffee enema can be very helpful in speeding up the detoxification process.

Coffee enemas can help to:

- Detoxify and heal the colon and the liver
- Open up the bile ducts and help to increase the production of bile
- Reduce different types of pain
- Reduce or eliminate many symptoms of toxicity from

disease conditions, and during healing crises
- Reduce parasites in the colon and liver
- Increase mental clarity, improve moods, increase feelings of energy, and improve digestion.

Colonics

Colonics are basically large-volume enemas, using many quarts of water at each session to gently and thoroughly cleanse the entire large intestine. Water is injected through a tube that has been inserted into the rectum. Then several ounces are allowed to be expelled, carrying wastes from the colon with it. This procedure is usually carried out by a colon therapist and lasts from thirty to sixty minutes. The process is not uncomfortable. After two or three colonics the rejuvenation benefits are usually quite evident. In addition to removing poisons, colonics exercise colon muscles, help to reshape your colon and stimulate colon reflex points that relate to other organs and parts of your body.

Colonic irrigations are safe and have been practiced for hundreds of years. Present-day fears about colon therapy are based on misinformation.

Some people who are serious about staying young and healthy have colon therapy units in their homes and perform them two or three times every week. By doing this and by eating properly, acid conditions never have a chance of building up in their systems. The resulting benefits are increased energy, better skin, less wrinkles, improved digestion, and improved bowel function. The benefits are systemic, meaning all functions in your body are improved.

Dr. Norman Walker, who was an early natural treatment

doctor, lived an active life until he died at the age of 109. He was strongly in favor of colon cleansing. He recommended using colonics on a regular basis to keep the colon clean. However, we can also use enemas to help this process.

Other ways to help your body detoxify

There are many things we can do to help our bodies detoxify, but I will mention three important ones:

- Saunas
- Walking and rebounding
- Safe fasting.

Saunas

Saunas cause the body temperature to rise and sweat is produced as part of the body's temperature control. During this process, toxins are released from tissues near the surface of the skin and eliminated from the body along with the perspiration.

Walking, rebounding, and vibrating

Walking, swimming, or any other activity that increases heart rate for a continuous period of twenty to forty minutes is good exercise. Without regular movement your body cannot be really healthy. The best and most efficient overall exercise is five to fifteen minutes each day on a rebounder or mini-trampoline. Because it utilizes the rapid reversal of gravity, every cell in your body is exercised, which improves blood circulation and lymphatic movement for the elimination of cellular wastes. Most whole-body vibrators also do this. Remember that your lymphatic system depends on body muscle movement to be able to transport wastes to your liver for processing out of your body.

Safe fasting

Fasting is the deliberate creation of conditions that allow your body an opportunity to restore itself to its original state of excellence. It gives our digestive systems and organs a rest from having to process a continual load of food. Your body cannot be fed solid food and detoxify at the same time. Fresh raw low-sweet fruit and vegetable juices are the exception.

Fasting is often the only way our bodies can detoxify quickly enough in cases of chronic disease. It is also useful as a means of preventing illness. During fasting it is helpful to have an enema each day to remove the released toxins from your body quickly.

There are many fasting regimens and they all have their merits. However, from research and my own personal experience I do not recommend water fasting. I believe it is important to give your body raw fresh low-sweet fruit and vegetable juices, which allow it to gain nutrients from them while being able to continue removing wastes from tissues, glands, and organs. Two of my favorite fasts are the watermelon fast and the Master Cleanse.[50]

An easy and very effective fast that extends the time each day when your body is naturally detoxifying is to not eat any cooked food or drink coffee until later in the morning or

---

50 Burroughs, Stanley. *The Master Cleanse*. http://ifayomi.com/assets/TheMasterCleanse.pdf

until noon. The meaning of breakfast is 'breaking the fast,' because during the night without having to process food your body is naturally working to cleanse itself internally. This works best when a person does not eat after the dinner meal. As soon as we eat cooked food or drink coffee for instance, our body has to switch over from cleaning out to processing again. Raw fruit, vegetables, and their freshly made juices do not break this fast. By doing this you are giving your body an extra few hours to clean out. Over time, after an initial adjustment period you will begin to notice that you start to feel lighter and have more energy. And the benefits of this practice continue the longer you are able to make it a habit.

Fasts are usually done for anywhere from one day to a week before returning to a regular diet. However, it is very important to break a fast properly as you move on to eating solid food again. During a fast the organs of digestion and assimilation are mostly at rest. They are not producing and secreting the usual amounts of digestive juices and enzymes. If solid food, and especially cooked food, is taken soon after a fast it can be a shock to your body and can cause problems with digestion. Your system needs to be gently encouraged back into action by starting with broths and soups, then salads, and finally meals with solid foods.

Bath soaks

During the period when you are attempting to correct an acid pH condition, it is also very helpful to have regular soaks in the bathtub. Three or more 30- to 40-minute baths per week can be taken in very warm to mildly hot water to which two or three handfuls of crystallized sea salt, Epsom salts, or a cup of food-grade hydrogen peroxide have been added. Afterward, towel dry but do not shower off.

The advantages of these soak-baths are twofold: one, toxins are drawn out of your body; and two, alkaline minerals from the salts, or oxygen from hydrogen peroxide, are absorbed into your body to increase its alkaline reserves and energy.

Liver cleansing

Your liver is the master organ and gland in your body; it performs over six hundred functions. If your liver is not clean – free of congestion, it cannot operate properly. It would be like a car radiator that cannot cool the engine water because it is clogged and corroded; it needs to be flushed. Similarly, your liver may need to be cleansed several times to increase its overall efficiency. Acid wastes that are stored in tissues, joints, and fat layers cannot be disposed of as long as your colon and your liver are congested and under-functioning. As mentioned previously, coffee retention enemas help with this, but the occasional liver flush is more intensive.

Going through a liver flush to remove stones, which are made up of mostly cholesterol crystals, from the liver and gallbladder may be the most difficult and 'not fun' procedure we will undertake on the road to improved health, yet it is necessary if we want to slow and reverse the aging process. As we get used to the routine it isn't all that bad. According to many practitioners, although it may be somewhat unpleasant it is absolutely safe. However, one must not attempt this cleanse when seriously ill because the body does use a significant amount of energy in the process.

There are several different approaches to cleansing the liver. Essentially, what is involved is reducing the strain on the liver by eliminating red meats, concentrated fats, and refined foods, as well as consuming liquids and herbs for a few days to soften deposits in the liver. Then on the evening before the flush, drink a mixture of fresh lemon juice and olive oil, and go directly to bed and lie as still as possible for the night. An Epsom salts drink in the morning is also part of this regimen. Later in the morning, stones of various sizes should be eliminated in several bowel movements.

A gentle liver detox kit may be found on Dr. Linda Page's website online.[51] A more aggressive recipe for liver and gallbladder flushes may be found under the name of Dr. Hulda Clark, online.[52]

Removing heavy metals from the body

As indicated in the previous chapter, heavy metals present a serious drain on our health and they have become pervasive in our present environment. We take them into our bodies from various sources including: air polluted by smoke and fuel exhausts, contaminated water, cigarettes, dental fillings, cooking utensils, vaccinations, cosmetics, household cleaners, plastics, and industrial activities such as hydrogenation of food products, electroplating and arc welding – to name a few.

---

51 www.healthyhealing.com/dr-lindas-blog/are-you-ready-for-a-liver-detox

52 www.drclark.net/cleanses/advanced/liver-cleanse-page/liver-cleanse-recipe

Removing these poisons from the body is not easy but it must be done to become truly healthy. It takes knowledge of how to do it and persistence in staying with a heavy metal detoxification program. It needs to be a lifetime and lifestyle endeavour because we are continually being exposed to these metals on an ongoing basis. Due to space constraints in this book, I will touch only on the main aspects of heavy metal detoxification and leave you to pursue further details about effective protocols online or in other books.

Foods known to help in eliminating heavy metals from the body include: pectin from rinds of fruits, cilantro, parsley, sulphur-rich foods such as onions and garlic, and chlorella. However, for deeply embedded heavy metal storage in the body, one will probably need a more aggressive approach. Effective products to do this include liquid zeolite and French green clay. The latter is known to be very effective in removing heavy metals and radiation from the body when taken over a period of time, although very little is known about this product in North America.[53] Please go online to research how to properly use these products.

HELPING YOUR BODY

We have covered a lot of information in this chapter and I emphasize again that you don't have to do it all at once. Take your time. Pick what you are comfortable with and work on that. Then as time goes by, gradually introduce

---

53   Hull, Janet Starr. PhD. *The Secret Of My French Green Clay - What I Learned From The Soviets*. http://bit.ly/1m7Z8DV

more of the practices that will help your body build better health.

I have talked about some major negative practices that we need to start correcting first, followed by what we can expect as our body starts to gain enough energy and nutrition to throw out the bad stuff in our bodies and begin to repair and renew itself. I talked about how long it can take to start feeling better and eventually regain full and vibrant health. And finally, I discussed the subject of detoxification and some ways it can be done.

Now in case you are wondering if changing your lifestyle to what I am suggesting is worth the effort, let me leave you with this thought: If you are a person who is eating the standard American diet and is doing many of the harmful health practices I have talked about in the second and third chapters, think about what the statistics are saying could be waiting for you in your health (or disease) future. We now know that unless your body is fed proper nutrients and helped to eliminate its wastes and toxins on a regular basis, it *will* develop various disease conditions eventually. That's not a *maybe* – it is a *will happen* situation.

Serious conditions such as diabetes, arthritis, heart disease, strokes, and cancer don't just happen all of a sudden for no reason. They have been developing for many years before you know something is wrong and medical science can diagnose them. By then we are talking about serious lifestyle restrictions and probably suffering, or even heroic efforts to save your life for a few more years. So here is the thing I really want you to think about. Again, *if* your present lifestyle is one that is harmful to your health, a serious disease condition could be developing in your body right now. Wouldn't it be wise to help your body turn the disease bus around while you have time and can still be in control? If you do this, you can really change the odds in your favor.

Prescription drugs

A word of caution is needed for those who are on medications under a doctor's supervision. Some medications require a long withdrawal period. Please consult with your doctor before reducing or stopping your use of prescription drugs.

In the next chapter I will talk about a subject that is rarely included in other health books and programs. But it is so important that if it is not addressed it can, and often does, block your body's ability to heal.

CHAPTER 5

ATTITUDES, EMOTIONS AND BELIEFS

Who or what is directing your life?

Have you ever wondered why things in your life keep happening the way they do? Even though you keep trying or praying or hoping for things to change for the better, it's pretty much the same? Frustrating isn't it? For some people, this chapter could be the breakthrough they have been looking for. Once we are able to understand why things happen to us the way they do and how to deal with our unresolved pain from negative emotional experiences, we can get our lives moving on a positive track again.

This chapter is a departure from foods, toxins, and the chemistry of health. It is about the silent controller behind the scenes that is directing *everything* in our lives. Even though we don't realize it, most of what happens to us and the effect it has on our health is created by our thought patterns and emotions, which come from our underlying subconscious beliefs.

Most people think that how they think or believe has little to do with their health or a disease they might have. However, recent research and the experience of alternative health practitioners is proving quite the opposite. I am going to present some background information on how our attitudes actually create and run our lives, and therefore have a great influence on the health we have or the diseases we want to be rid of. Attitudes and beliefs can be the reason why some people can't lose weight or overcome major illnesses such as cancer, even though they have gone through all the diets, treatments, and therapy. Something is holding back the change they want.

What some natural treatment doctors are saying

When I first started to study natural health under the guidance of Dr. Joel Robbins, he had a saying that went like this: "If you can't get rid of your attitude problem, you are not going to get rid of your physical problem." Wow! That was a wake-up thought for me.

More recently, when listening to alternative cancer doctors, such as Dr. Nicholas Gonzales and others talking about how to overcome serious disease, I heard them say that, in addition to very good nutrition, enzyme therapy, and detoxification, the other factor that *must be addressed and corrected* is attitude. If people cannot move into a positive frame of mind, they will not be able to overcome disease. Recovering your health *depends* on a reassessment and overhaul of the attitudes and beliefs you have.

BASIC UNDERSTANDING

In the first chapter I said that we need to be *aware* or *conscious* of everything that is either building or destroying our health. Most of us concentrate on being aware of what we are eating or drinking and knowing whether these are good or bad for us. *However*, and this is a *big* however, don't underestimate what your mind is doing to you! Let's start by realizing that we have two minds: the conscious mind and the subconscious mind.

The conscious mind

The conscious mind is the mind we are aware of. It is the tool we use to think with. This is the part of us we use to express our personality. It has the ability to think about the past, present, and future. It also gives us the ability to judge, assess facts, and make choices. The conscious mind is the foundation of our free will. It is active when we are awake, but there is another mind that takes over when we sleep, and also works automatically behind the scenes when we are awake. It is the real powerhouse and silent controller and director of our lives. It is…

The subconscious mind

We may think that our conscious thoughts are in control while we are awake, but the subconscious mind directs even our *thinking*, from behind the scenes, despite the fact that we are not aware of it. It is the real brains behind *how* we think because it has been programmed by our life experiences – the good things and the bad things that happen to us. Still, the subconscious mind only works in the present. It doesn't make judgments; it just responds to the programming of our core beliefs, the same way a computer program responds to the software codes written for it. That's why it is important for us to examine and become aware of our deeply-held beliefs about the major things in our life such as money, relationships, learning, spirituality, and health.

The subconscious mind allows us to operate automatically in activities such as breathing, driving a car, or pulling our hands away from a hot stove. It can also sort through the huge amount of information stored in our memory bank to help us solve problems, make plans, and find something we have misplaced. But until we have changed our core beliefs, our subconscious mind also causes us to repeatedly do things we vowed not to, such as going into losing investments again and again, gambling, smoking, drinking too much alcohol, or attracting the same kind of negative personal relationships into our lives. The subconscious mind is like a super computer; it is an *amazing* resource. But the key to our happiness is to make sure it is programmed for positive outcomes in our life.

Our negative emotional charge

Painful experiences from childhood, reinforced by other emotional hurts at a later stage in life, build up within us as a negative emotional charge that sits in our subconscious mind, blocking our ability to experience full happiness, success, and joy. It takes over our life, coloring our view of everything and preventing the development of true intimacy in our relationships. This negative emotional charge can show up in personality traits such as: a pessimistic attitude, being sarcastic, controlling, manipulative, critical, being super-sensitive, taking offense, becoming angry, raging, blaming, feeling that one is a victim, lacking self-worth, and *expecting* to be short-changed in the abundance and happiness that other people seem to enjoy. We can develop a poverty complex or a persecution complex, which keeps those things re-occurring in our lives.

In some cases our emotional pain was caused in the past by circumstances beyond our control. For example, as children we have no control of the family we were born into, or the house and neighbourhood we lived in, or the food or protection we were given. We should not feel guilty or think these things were our fault; we were not the cause of them. Once we become aware of old unresolved pain, we need to acknowledge it, accept it, and work to release it, so that our life can get moving on a positive track again.

Eckhart Tolle, author of *The Power of Now*, calls these painful experiences a negative energy field. It occupies our attention, causing us to identify with the pain as part of who we are. When this happens, we lose touch with who we really are as loving beings. This causes a great conflict inside us because we are not viewing ourselves holistically. As a result, we try to run from the emotional discomfort. We don't want to feel pain, so we turn to methods of sedation, like drugs and alcohol or eating too much; we try to escape. We do not know how to heal the conflict so we continue to live *unconsciously,* as if we are on auto-pilot. But love, joy, and peace cannot really blossom until you have freed yourself from the control of your mind – the painful thoughts that keep going round and round in your head, like a hamster on a wheel. The true person you are is a loving spirit, just as every little baby is when it is born. You need to be in contact with this loving spirit again.

The purpose of emotional pain

Emotional pain is an imbalance of emotions, which confuses our ability to see *objectively* and clearly. Emotion is e-motion, which *means* energy in motion. Our emotional energy is meant to flow freely. When it becomes blocked or stuck, it can lead to poor health and disease as well as all the discomfort and unhappiness that go along with it.

One of my all-time favorite books, which I have owned since I was twenty years old, is Kahlil Gibran's 1923 masterpiece, *The Prophet*. In a beautiful poetical style, the Prophet shares his wisdom with others on life's common experiences and challenges. When a woman asks him to speak of pain he says: "Your pain is the breaking of the shell that encloses your understanding." To me, that statement is so profound and so meaningful, because it opened up the idea for me that pain has a purpose.

When we experience and recognize our pain rather than try to block it out, it can lead us to an understanding of the emotional part of us that is crying to be recognized and healed. The purpose of emotional pain is to attract our attention so we can work to change our thinking, our beliefs, and our habits. The same applies to much of our physical pain; it is a cry for attention to change something in our life.

TAKING CONTROL

When we learn to notice and listen to our thoughts, we are in the present moment; we have moved into awareness and control. All that chatter in our mind is always about the past or the future, but the past is only a memory and the future is only imaginings. As long as we are rehearsing stressful memories we cannot move forward into health, peace, and true happiness. You cannot change the past no matter how hard you try. The present moment is the only opportunity to bring about change. The present moment is the only reality and that is where your power is. Living in the present NOW is where peace is found. And here is a wonderful truth – we can learn to tell our minds what to focus on.

Once we do this, we are able to control our minds and direct our thoughts, and we naturally begin to feel more confident, peaceful, and in control. Once we are aware of our thoughts, the next step is to become aware of the feelings that are generated by our thoughts because our feelings create our attitudes and emotions. And *they* really run our lives.

Attitudes

Our attitudes shape who we are; they form our character. They are formed from our beliefs and they become the steering wheels of our lives. If we have an open heart and a teachable mind we will be continually learning and improving our character. If we have a closed mind or negative outlook on life we will tend to lock out opportunities for learning and character improvements, and remain stuck in the past. Because you are reading this right now, it means that you are open to learning something new that you may not have known before; you are opening your mind to the possibility of positive growth.

Emotions

Emotions are strong generalized feelings that have both psychological and physiological effects. Strong emotions produce chemicals in our bodies that have definite influences on our health. For example, remember how happy and energetic you felt when you were first in love. On the other hand, when you are sad or depressed you have a hard time dragging yourself out of bed in the morning; you feel tired and lack motivation to get going and tackle jobs that need to be done.

The emotional reaction we have to any experience is *directly related* to our thoughts about it. Are our thoughts happy, hopeful, loving, sad, hateful, fearful, or angry? It is our *perception* of events, how we are viewing them, that determines what we feel. We *know* the feelings of emotion such as anger for example, but often we are not aware that the anger is coming from *unresolved* emotional pain. Our buttons get pushed and we don't understand why; we just react. We might fly off the handle with outbursts of anger or maybe crying. We may think someone else is doing it to us, but it is our own attitudes and thoughts about what they say or do that trigger our unresolved pain and cause our emotional responses. If we are not aware of our emotions, we are like a ship without a rudder, tossed about by the winds of circumstances in our lives.

Our emotional experiences are created by how we talk to ourselves in our head. Instead of blocking out our painful emotions with outbursts of anger, submission, continual activity, addictive substances, or going to the fridge, we need to become aware of our emotions *as they are happening* and work to resolve our pain. An example might be of a person who lost his loving partner in a fatal car accident. Instead of working through the process of healing from the grief, he distracts himself with continual activity, very little sleep, and too much alcohol. This avoidance of the natural emotional healing process only suppresses pain and sets the stage for serious disease such as heart problems or cancer, at a later date.

When we have emotional pain it is our body talking to us, trying to get our attention to help us become whole again, to come into balance. We need to understand its language, pay attention to it, and do something about the emotional pain because it is affecting the health of our body.

Negative attitudes and emotions are not fun. We do not like having them and we do not like being around those who display them. When *we* are being negative or are near a negative person, we feel like putting up our defences. This emotional reaction has an effect in our physical bodies. We operate the same way on a cellular level.

Research by cellular biologist Dr. Bruce Lipton has totally changed conventional views on how cells work. Cells don't just operate from the inside-out, taking direction from their genes; they work from the outside-in, taking direction from their emotional and chemical environments. Each cell's membrane, or 'mem-brain' as he calls it, senses what the cell *needs* to be able to grow and survive from its environment, and then gives direction to the proteins inside it.

Dr. Lipton has shown that each cell has intelligence and that what applies to one cell also applies to groups of cells. Your body is a community of 70 trillion or more cells; it is a huge collection of cellular intelligence. In his book *The Biology of Belief*, Dr. Lipton explains that cells are either growing or protecting themselves. When cells sense nutrition in their environment, they move toward it for growth. When they sense a threat to their well-being, they go into protection mode and move away. We do the same.

When we are newly born we naturally respond to good nutrition and love; we feel energized and supported, and start to grow. But when the receptors in our bodies sense toxins or chemicals or emotions that cause *fear*, we go into protection mode; we retreat and stop growing. Our physical body senses threats through the hypothalamus gland in the head, which sends a message to the master gland, the pituitary, which then signals the adrenal glands to release the stress hormone adrenaline. Adrenaline starts a fight or flight response. In the interest of survival, this diverts blood flow from the internal organs and brain to the muscles. We speed up and move to a state of high tension. Digestion and internal nourishment, plus the ability to think intelligently, take a back seat to brute strength. During this time our immune system is suppressed. We become physically stronger, but intellectually weaker; we are in protection mode.

The critical point to understand is that positive emotions help us thrive and grow, while negative emotions cause us to just survive; they hold us back from growing.

The two basic emotions – Love and Fear

Our emotions have a purpose. Positive emotions and attitudes such as joy, hope, optimism, contentment, and gratitude are based in love and make us feel good about ourselves. We feel alive and open. We develop a positive self-image and we grow. Negative emotions such as anger, resentment, guilt, anxiety, and depression have their basis in fear and in feelings of powerlessness and lack of self-worth. Under the influence of negative emotions we feel vulnerable and put up our defences. Negative emotions stunt our growth. Love encourages us to grow. Fear discourages us and causes us to move into protection mode; we shrink back into ourselves. Love promotes health and energy generation, while fear promotes dis-ease and energy depletion.

Negative emotions exert a drain on a person's cardio-vascular, immune, and hormonal systems, whereas positive emotions have a rewarding and regenerative effect on these same systems.[54] The whole body works better under the influence of positive emotions.

LINKING EMOTIONS TO THE CHEMISTRY OF HEALTH

The chemical by-product of a negative emotional stress response in our bodies is acid. As we have learned, acidic conditions create an environment for disease. That's why we need to be conscious of our negative emotional habits so we can work to change them to positive attitudes that have an alkalizing effect in our body. When you move to positive attitudes, you relieve your body of stress and help it to produce health.

---

54   Childre, Doc; Martin, Howard; Beech, Donna. *The Heartmath Solution*. HarperCollins Publishers. 1999. p. 19.

Negative attitudes work against healing, even though they appear to give temporary satisfaction or relief when we express them. Reacting to situations with anger, fear, worry, grief, or apathy, causes a lack of ease in our bodies. This is because the energy of our thoughts, beliefs, and attitudes is connected to our organs through energy pathways. When we continue to allow a negative view of the world to dominate our thinking, it results in small changes in energy flow to organs. Over time, this restricted energy results in cellular changes and function which, in turn, leads to the development of disease. By the time doctors and medical technology can identify a disease in the body it is well advanced. By then in order to heal, in addition to intensive detoxification and healthy nutrition, we must work to identify the emotional blockages and release them so that the disease bus can be completely turned around.

When we take responsibility for our thoughts and build attitudes of acceptance, gratitude, generosity, forgiveness, humility, and love into our thinking and actions, the negative aspects of our character, such as selfishness, bitterness, guilt, regret, and self-condemnation begin to lose their power and start to disappear. When we do this, we are reprogramming our subconscious mind; we are moving from being self-centered to being other-centered. We are learning to live in the present moment. We are learning to live in peace and harmony with our self. And when upsets do come into our life, we can recognize them for what they are – a signal or opportunity to check on the state of our thoughts, attitudes, emotions, and beliefs.

Unlike negative thoughts and emotions, positive thoughts and emotions have a calming, healing, and regenerative effect on the whole body. Attitudes of happiness, gratitude, thankfulness, love, forgiveness, patience, and so forth, are relaxing, stress-reducing, and are supportive to all body functions. Laughter is especially healing – so much so that many hospitals in America now incorporate humour therapy along with traditional treatments for injuries and diseases such as cancer.[55] Laughter has been found to lower the body's cortisol (stress-induced chemical) levels, and strengthen the immune system.[56] Take the opportunity to laugh as much as you can.

Whatever we do, whether it is eating, working, or playing, should be done with thankfulness and love. Both attitudes play large roles in our emotional well-being. Thankfulness is a feeling of gratitude and appreciation. And although we are most familiar with feeling love as an emotion, in its pure form love is a way of *being* and relating to the world; it is an attitude. An attitude of love has all the qualities of acceptance, allowing, giving, sharing, and wishing the best for another person. It is the basis for peace and emotional stability in our lives.

Gratitude and love are the keys to harmony, not only in our relationships with people, but in our relationship to the food and beverages we consume. This is because our thoughts are energy, and as such they influence everything around us and even beyond.

---

55 Vogt, Victoria. *Can Laughter Cure Illness?* http://bit.ly/1nmc1x4

56 Ibid

Being authentic and real

We all have an inner sense of whether someone is being real or not. When we are being real we are authentic and genuine. There is no acting; our true self is coming across. Our authentic self is honest, open, and straightforward; it is free of ego – a preoccupation with self, as in pride, selfishness, or conceit. When we are authentic, we don't try to be anything other than who we are; we are transparent. Our authentic self is like a little child, always spontaneously natural and in the present moment. It has no agenda other than being who it is. Being our authentic self opens the door to truth, happiness, fulfillment, and joy in our lives. This helps us learn again who we are as a being of loving intent in all we say and do. It is who we were created to be. If we are not there yet, I believe it is who we came here on earth to become.

Getting our act together

Reshaping our character requires an honest examination and identification of both the positive and negative attitudes that operate in our lives. It means becoming aware that attitudes and emotions influence our health. It means taking responsibility for our attitudes and making the commitment to change the negative ones. No matter what attitudes our parents, friends, or associates influenced us with, or what our life experiences have been, as adults we are still responsible for our *own* attitudes. And, we are the only ones who can change them. Blaming others gets us nowhere except into a rut. Taking personal responsibility for where we are in life is the way to start improving our attitudes.

Healing on the mental/emotional side comes from being grateful and forgiving, as well as accepting responsibility for the consequences of our own decisions and actions. It is when we run into difficulties that we should be asking ourselves: "What can I learn from this? What am I doing wrong that should be changed?" Challenges and setbacks are opportunities to change our attitudes and beliefs for better outcomes in our lives.

Now what about beliefs? Why does our life unfold the way it does? Is there something that drives our life in the same direction it has been going for many years? When we say we want to change, and even make resolutions, why do some of us seem helpless to carry through and achieve different outcomes in our lives? For some of us it's the same old, same old. But why? There *is* an answer, and it all depends on what we believe.

BELIEFS RULE OUR LIVES

A long time ago, Henry Ford said: "Whether you think you can or you think you can't, you're right." Our beliefs are so powerful that they create our health, our happiness, and our lives. The beliefs we hold in our subconscious minds, whether positive or negative, are reflected in our life circumstances.

Every disease is connected to a false belief system within us about some aspect of our lives. Our bodies are talking to us and showing us. A disease process is evidence that something is wrong in the workings of the mind, and that is where the power to make lasting change is. The disease distress is our body's cry asking us to change the underlying cause which is the beliefs that are not working for the best in our life. In many cases it could just be the accepted beliefs we have about the food we eat.

Research by Dr. Bruce Lipton, mentioned earlier, proved that the biology of our cells is controlled by our minds. This is mainly because our thoughts, which stem from our beliefs, cause a different chemical response in our bodies depending on whether we feel safe or threatened, happy or annoyed, positive or negative. By sensing through their receptors, cells react to their environment by either growing or being protective. A healthy environment encourages a growth response, and a toxic environment causes your body to react with a protective response. It is the difference between healing and growing, or just surviving as best it can.

It is not necessarily what is true, but what we believe to be true – our perception – which is important. It is now becoming a proven reality in studies on the placebo effect that our minds can heal our bodies. There have been television documentaries on how people have been healed completely when they truly believed that a repairing-surgery had been performed or that a certain healing-medication had been administered, even though the surgery wasn't performed and the medication was just a sugar pill. Dr. Lipton said it really disturbs the pharmaceutical manufacturers that in *most* of their clinical trials, the placebos, the 'fake drugs,' prove to be just as effective as the engineered chemical cocktails.

The Bottom Line

The mind is very powerful. When our minds believe something to be true, this causes our bodies to respond and make it happen. We have all seen performances or programs where people are hypnotized and because they were told by the hypnotist that they would respond in a certain way, they did. This is because the hypnotist was able to program the person's subconscious mind when they were deeply relaxed, to believe a certain thing and they acted accordingly. This implanted belief told their brains and bodies how to behave and react.

This chapter was totally devoted to an examination of the role that our attitudes, emotions, and beliefs play in our mental and physical health. At the beginning of this chapter I told you that some health practitioners are finding that, without a positive attitude most people cannot recover from serious disease conditions. Becoming aware of our attitudes and underlying beliefs, and changing the ones that are not working for our best outcomes in our lives, are important parts of becoming healthy and staying that way.

In the next chapter I will focus on some common beliefs concerning health and treatments of disease that are deceiving us. They are deceptions, myths, half-truths, or lies. Consequently, they do more to harm our health than to build it. In my opinion, these deceptions are making millions of people sick.

CHAPTER 6

DECEPTIONS AND LIES

"It's not what we don't know that hurts.
It's what we know that ain't so."
– Will Rogers

We live in a commercial world where the goal of corporations and the people running them is to make money. The objective of promoting the health of individuals all too often takes second place.

We are influenced by family habits, cultural customs, and advertising to view most commercial foods as desirable and acceptable, that it doesn't matter what we eat as long as it tastes good and is convenient to make. Learning what might be healthy for you is mostly a hit-and-miss situation; one really has to think about it and 'dig' to learn how to keep one's body healthy. This often requires that we keep an open mind to be able to question accepted beliefs about health, nutrition, and medical practices. Conventional medical doctors offer little help in educating us about proper nutrition; they are mostly trained to identify diseases, not to teach patients how to stay healthy by eating foods that nourish their bodies. Further, the conventional medical system is firmly linked to and controlled by the pharmaceutical industry – the more drugs they sell, the more money they make. Their main focus is on treating disease symptoms with drugs. Drugs often create other side effects, which require additional treatment with other drugs. The end result is that customers and profits increase, but the causes of the diseases are not fully addressed and corrected.

In this chapter I am going to tell you about four major health deceptions, half-truths, or lies. They are part of the commercial brainwashing and misinformation the medical and food industries have bought into and promote. When we buy into them and accept them as truth, we are placing great hardships on our bodies and inviting health problems into our lives. When you understand the truth behind these deceptions you will be in a position to make more informed decisions for health improvements in your own life.

Deception #1 – Fat makes you fat

There is a popular belief that eating fat makes you fat. We are also told that fat causes heart attacks and that margarine is better for you than butter. These statements are either false or only half the story. They are deceptions. The push to get people to eat low-fat diets and choose low- or no-fat foods can be outright unhealthy. The truth is that the *wrong* kinds of fats are bad for you. Udo Erasmus, author of *Fats that Heal, Fats that Kill*, says that:

> Degenerative diseases that involve fats prematurely kill
> over two-thirds of the people currently living in affluent,
> industrialized nations. ... These deaths are the result of
> eating habits based on ignorance and misconceptions.[57]

Dr. Weston Price was a dentist and medical researcher in
Cleveland, Ohio. He conducted extensive research into the
relationship between nutrition, dental health, and physical
health. Early in the last century he travelled around the
world visiting isolated groups of people to study their diets.
What he found was that all groups were healthy on their
natural diets. They all ate some animal products. When he
analyzed the nutrient content of native diets he found that
they provided about ten times more fat-soluble vitamins
than the American diet of the 1930s. Since then, the
average American diet has included even less of the good
fats but so many more of the processed fats.

Many people today eat either the wrong kinds of
fats, or do not eat enough of the good fats to keep their
bodies healthy. The truth is that your body *depends* on a
regular supply of *good fats* and oils to build healthy cell
membranes and hormones. It also uses fat as its preferred
source of stored energy for sustained use throughout the
day.[58] Fat provides more than twice the energy that is

----

57   Erasmus, Udo, PhD. *Fats that Heal, Fats that Kill*. Alive Books, Burnaby
     BC Canada. 1994. p. 3.

58   *What Does it Mean to be Fat-Adapted?* www.marksdailyapple.com/what-
     does-it-mean-to-be-fat-adapted/#axzz2wFjY4T9G

available from carbohydrates.[59] In addition, the conversion of carbohydrates or protein into fat is about ten times less efficient than simply storing fat in a fat cell for later use.[60]

If your diet is loaded with bad fats, your body can only make low-quality cell membranes that don't function very well. Margarine is a good example of this because it is far from being a natural food. It is made from poor quality oils to begin with, by processing at high temperatures. It has nickel, emulsifiers, bleach and synthetic colors added, and it is hydrogenated. The final product has no nutritional value, does not rot, flies won't land on it, and nothing will grow on it. Sounds yummy doesn't it?

What kind of cell membranes do you think your body is able to make with that stuff? Margarine is a very bad fat.

Bad fats

When healthful natural oils from vegetables, fruits, seeds, or nuts are processed with high heat, metal catalysts, and hydrogenation, bad fats (for the body) are produced. These fats contain what are called trans-fatty acids, so-called because the processing 'transforms' an oil molecule from its natural state into a twisted, unnatural configuration. This may sound like a minor change in order to produce products that are cheaper and stay on store shelves for a long time without spoiling. "However, the results of this miniscule

---

59 *Carbohydrates vs Fats.* http://dl.clackamas.cc.or.us/ch106-07/carbohyd1. htm

60 Fruedenrich, Craig, PhD. *How Fat Cells Work.* http://science. howstuffworks.com/life/cellular-microscopic/fat-cell2.htm

change are drastic."[61] When trans-fats are consumed, the body doesn't recognize them or know how to use them; they are in a very real sense, artificial. Whereas natural oils are liquid at body and room temperatures, trans-fats are solid and sticky. Some health implications of trans- fats include:

- Blood platelets become more sticky, contributing to circulatory and cardiovascular problems
- Reduction of the rate at which enzymes can break down fatty acids, which in turn impairs the ability of the heart to function efficiently
- Weakening of the protective barrier around cells, making them more permeable – with holes in them – so that molecules that should be kept out may enter (causing allergic reactions), and molecules that should remain in cells can escape
- Reduction of energy flow and electrical efficiency within the body
- Interference with the body's inflammation response and immune system competence.[62]

The process of producing trans-fats, including home frying and deep-frying at high temperatures, also destroys the nutritional value of oils. When you fry foods, the best oils to use at low-to-medium temperatures are butter and coconut oil. Better yet, is to simmer food in water and then add good oil at a later stage.

---

61   Erasmus, Udo. Op. cit. p. 107.

62   Ibid. pp. 109, 110.

Examples of bad fat products are:

- Margarine and shortening (cheaper substitutes for butter and lard, respectively)
- Fats used in deep-frying
- Oils that have been hydrogenated, which unfortunately includes most of the oils on store shelves, such as Canola oil. Hydrogenation is a process that introduces hydrogen gas into oils under high pressure in the presence of a metal catalyst. Industry does this to produce "cheap spreadable (plastic) products for (non-discriminating) consumers, or to provide shelf stability at the expense of nutritional value.[63]" They are referred to as plastic or near-plastic because when oil is hydrogenated to create trans fat, it creates a plastic-like substance with a melting point of 112 degrees Fahrenheit (44.5°C).[64] (Butter is a good natural fat with a melting point beginning at approximately 85 degrees Fahrenheit (28°C).
- Processed cheese
- Processed peanut butter
- French fries
- Candies
- Cookies.

Good fats

Good oils (fats) for the body are the essential fatty acids and

63   Ibid. p. 100.

64   *The Toxic Truth About Trans Fat.* http://transformative-nutrition.com/resources/articles/the-toxic-truth-about-trans-fat/

unsaturated fats. Essential fatty acids (EFAs) are necessary fats that humans cannot synthesize within their bodies; they are obtained through diet. They are more commonly known as omega-3 and omega-6 fatty acids. Essential fatty acids are utilized by the body to build cell structure, to help generate electrical energy, and produce hormones. They are required for nerve impulses, brain development and function, healthy skin, digestion, inner organ function, the cardiovascular system, and immune system. They are critically important for health. Most people are oil deficient because good oils are lacking in their diets.

All the essential fatty acids are obtained from a diet of natural unprocessed food. Examples of essential fatty acid oils which one can supplement their diet with are: hempseed oil and flaxseed oil.

Unsaturated oils, or unsaturated fats as they are sometimes referred to, are liquid at room temperature. They are so named because they lack two or more hydrogen atoms in their molecular structure. Raw vegetables, fruits, grains, nuts, and seeds contain naturally-occurring unsaturated fats.

Saturated fats are so-called because they have no openings in their chemical structure. They are usually solid at room temperature. Naturally-occurring saturated fats are found mainly in animal fats, meats, dairy products, eggs, and tropical oils.

Saturated fats are also synthesized in the body from carbohydrates. Contrary to popular belief, not all saturated fats are responsible for the many diseases they are accused of contributing to. In fact, saturated fats are very necessary and are utilized by the body – for energy, to build cell membranes, for the incorporation of calcium into bone structure, and to strengthen the immune system. However, long-chain fatty acids, found mostly in animal and dairy products, do have a tendency to aggregate or stick together, causing sticky blood platelets. This is why people who consume large amounts of animal and dairy products suffer from an increased incidence of cardiovascular disease.

Unsaturated EFAs, like those found in seed oils and fish, prevent saturated fats from aggregating by keeping them dispersed. This may explain why Eskimos who consumed traditional diets had a very low incidence of heart disease. The fat of land animals does not contain omega-3 EFAs, whereas the fat of sea mammals and fish does.

Why does a body store fat?

This is a question that people trying to lose weight do not understand. Why a body becomes fat is not just about eating too many calories. It is also about eating foods that contain chemical additive toxins, and foods that upset the body's acid/alkaline balance.

Your body cannot completely digest and use unnatural incomplete foods. Its organs of elimination become congested – plugged-up and sluggish. And because of incomplete elimination, it is forced to store toxins away from vital organs and glands where they will cause the least harm. The body insulates toxins in fat to protect the rest of the body from their harmful effects.

What makes you fat is a diet containing an excess of refined carbohydrates, sugars, and artificial sweeteners.

They are nutrient-poor and lacking in fiber, allowing them to be digested and absorbed rapidly. Consequently, the body is flooded with excess glucose. In attempts to deal with this situation, the body either stores the glucose as fat, or spills it into our urine – a common sign of diabetes.[65] In summary, if your body is storing fat it is probably doing so because it has no choice; your diet lacks proper nutrition, fiber, water, healthy oils, and efficient elimination.

This next deception is also nutrition-related, but getting it right in your own health program is very important.

Deception #2 – Salt is bad for you

I talked briefly about this one in the third chapter but I am focussing on it again here because it is so important to make this change in your eating plan. Salt – the right kind, is *essential* for life. You can't live without it.

The statements that salt is bad for you or that sodium is bad for you are half-truths, because it is the wrong kind of salt – *table salt*, that is bad for you. This kind of salt is in most processed foods as well as on most of our kitchen tables.

Common *table salt*, or sodium chloride, is salt that has been refined, processed, and stripped of its minerals. It is toxic and addictive. Refined salt is a chemical compound that has no food value. It cannot be digested or assimilated because, from a chemistry point of view, the sodium and chlorine are so tightly bound together. It is inorganic or not alive, so your body cannot work with it. It builds up in

65   Ibid. p. 34

your body. It is very acidifying and leads to many disease conditions. It causes your body to hold on to extra water. It is harmful to your heart and has been linked to high blood pressure and hardening of the arteries. It places great stress on your kidneys and replaces calcium and potassium in your body, which can lead to osteoporosis and heart disease.

The real truth is that your body depends on proper salt to go on living. Did you know that in the Middle Ages salt was traded ounce for ounce for pure gold, because it was considered so important?[66] Without a properly-balanced salt base we run out of electrolytes and the cellular batteries in our bodies die out. Refined table salt, and even many of the processed sea salts available from health food stores, can promote calcification and a breakdown of cellular tissue.

Our blood needs natural whole salt to function because cells must be bathed in a sodium-based fluid. Digestion depends on having a sufficient quantity of stomach hydrochloric acid to properly digest proteins. Hydrochloric acid can only be produced if organic chlorine is available in the right ratio. The solution to these requirements can be found in whole natural sea salt. In addition, natural sea salt is a great source of at least 84 available minerals and trace minerals that our bodies need. You can find several varieties of unprocessed, natural sea salt in health food stores.

Table salt and its toxic chemical artificial cousins, such as monosodium glutamate (MSG), make us want to eat

---

66 Trentmann, Frank. *The Oxford Handbook of the History of Consumption*. Oxford University Press. 2012. p. 131.

and drink more. MSG is a processed, concentrated form of salt that is used as a flavor enhancer in thousands of food products. It is an excitotoxin, which means it over-excites cells to the point of damage or death. MSG induces serious nerve damage in the body.[67] But specific to our discussion here, when scientists want to fatten rats or mice for experiments, they inject or feed them with MSG.[68] MSG ingestion stimulates insulin secretion.[69] When it is fed to rats, it causes the rodents to become grossly obese. Do you think that might have something to do with why we humans gain weight and can't lose it? Check the labels on foods in your cupboards and on store shelves and you will find that MSG is in many of the canned and processed foods and fast foods we have been eating. To make it difficult for people to know what they are eating, MSG is also disguised by other names such as: autolyzed yeast, yeast extract, maltodextrin, hydrolyzed protein, sodium caseinate, mono-potassium glutamate, and textured protein.

In summary, looking back on the first two health myths regarding fat and salt, if these are the first changes you make as a start to your new lifestyle you will be taking two

---

67   Blaylock, Russel. L, MD. *Excitotoxins, the Taste that Kills*, Health Press. Santa Fe, NM. 1997.

68   Fenwick, Chuck. Director Medical Corps. *How Do You Make a Rat Fat? And what it means for you*. www.medicalcorps.org/fat-rat.htm

69   Graham, T. E; Sgro, V; Friars, D; Gibala, M. J. *Glutamate ingestion: the plasma and muscle free amino acid pools of resting humans*. American Journal of Physiology - Endocrinology and MetabolismPublished 1 January 2000Vol. 278no. E83-E89. http://ajpendo.physiology.org/content/278/1/E83.full

huge steps to improving your health. You are on your way.

The following two deceptions are medically-based, and this next one is huge!

Deception #3 – Cholesterol is bad for you

Whereas the first two deceptions about fat and salt are laced with half-truths, this one is an outright lie. There is so much information and research that explains and proves that this is so. When I started to research this subject I did a quick Google-search on the Internet, using various words. Here is what I found:

Cholesterol hoax	–	388,000 results
Cholesterol myth	–	2,000,000 results
Cholesterol lie	–	3,480,000 results
Cholesterol con	–	8,200,000 results

The evidence is overwhelming that our entire population has been duped into believing that cholesterol is the cause of heart disease and therefore, should be treated with cholesterol-lowering statin drugs. It has been a very successful deception from a drug sales point of view. Here is an example from the United States for 2013,

The cholesterol-lowering drug Crestor was the nation's most prescribed drug in the past 12 months, according to a new report from research firm IMS Health. New prescriptions and refills of the drug totaled 23.7 million.[70]

Statin drugs reduce cholesterol by blocking the liver enzyme responsible for making it, but they also interfere with other biological functions such as sex hormone and cortisone production, and they deplete the body of the energy nutrient CoQ10,[71] to cite a few of their side effects.

What we need to understand about cholesterol is that it is essential for life and the health of our entire body. The body manufactures cholesterol in the liver and in skin cells regardless of whether it is consumed in the diet or not. We do not need to obtain it from food. The body utilizes cholesterol to manufacture steroid hormones and vitamin D. Cholesterol is a component of all cells and is found in large amounts in nerve tissues and the brain. It is also required in various bodily tissue structures, is part of the process of fat digestion, and may at times serve as an antioxidant. It is also an essential part of the body's repair kit.

Where mainstream medicine got off-track with cholesterol and heart disease was when it was noticed that it was sometimes present, along with fats, the protein fibrin, and calcium in the arteries of people with heart disease.[72] However, what wasn't realized was that when arteries

---

70   WebMD. *Crestor Tops List of Best-Selling Drugs.* www.webmd.com/ cholesterol-management/news/20131101/crestor-is-top-selling-drug

71   Mercola, Joseph. *DO. Do You Take Any of These 11 Dangerous Statins or Cholesterol Lowering Drugs?* http://articles.mercola.com/sites/articles/ archive/2010/07/20/the-truth-about-statin-drugs-revealed.aspx

72   Erasmus, Udo, PhD. *Fats that Heal, Fats that Kill.* Alive Books, Burnaby BC Canada. 1994. p. 70.

become weakened due to a diet deficient in micronutrients, the body starts trying to repair the weakened walls by laying down a coating of cholesterol. If this continues over a long period of time it can lead to slower blood flow, heart attacks and strokes.[73] Of course, the problem is not cholesterol; it is nutrition – a diet deficient in minerals, proteins, and good oils which are needed to maintain tissue integrity. Too much sugar can also be a contributing factor:

> The real cause of heart disease is related to damage inflicted on the inside of your arteries, the primary culprit of which is sugar, which causes plaque formation and thickening of the artery wall.[74]

To further pop the cholesterol balloon is the fact that more people die of low cholesterol than of high cholesterol. That people with high cholesterol live the longest has been the conclusion of many scientific papers.[75] If we interfere with the body's cholesterol-making process, we are upsetting its natural efforts to repair and balance systems within our bodies. In time this can lead to many chronic disease conditions.

Try to remember that your body is wonderfully made. It doesn't do anything by mistake; everything is done for a

---

73   Niedzwiecki, Aleksandra. *Exposing the Cholesterol Fraud*. Dr. Rath Health Foundation. http://bit.ly/1lBKIiw

74   Mercola, Joseph. DO. Statin Nation: *The Great Cholesterol Coverup*. http://bit.ly/1esMDmr

75   Ravnskov, Uffe. MD. PhD. *The Cholesterol Myths - The Benefits of High Cholesterol*. www.ravnskov.nu/myth9.htm

reason. If it raises your cholesterol level, it does so because it is trying to correct something. If we interfere with this process, it is like turning off the power to one or more engines in an aircraft – sooner or later, a crash will happen. Your body will carry on as long as it can, but with fewer tools and weakened efficiency. Your job is to learn what it requires in the way of nutrition and lifestyle to be healthy, and try to supply that. When you do this, your body will work hard to reward you with good health – free of disease.

The last deception I will tell you about concerns the commonly accepted treatments for cancer, how misleading the information is, and how ineffective these treatments can be.

Deception #4 – Conventional cancer treatments

We are told by conventional medical authorities and members of the cancer industry that the most effective treatments for various cancers are chemotherapy and radiation. But is this true?

When patients are diagnosed with cancer, fear is often used to get them to undergo chemotherapy or radiation treatments. They are discouraged from seeking alternative treatments. Chemotherapy and radiation treatments are designed to kill cancer cells but unfortunately, other cells and the whole body suffer ill effects as well. Five year cancer survival rates are estimated to range from as low as 2.1%[76] to

---

76   Morgan, Graeme; Ward, Robin; Barton, Michael. *The Contribution of Cytotoxic Chemotherapy to 5-year Survival in Adult Malignancies.* Clinical Oncology, Volume 16, Issue 8, pp 549-560. 2004. http://www. clinicaloncologyonline.net/article/S0936-6555(04)00222-5/abstract

60% or more,[77] depending on the type and stage of a cancer, and other treatments used along with chemotherapy.

Surveys of oncologists show that 75% of world doctors would refuse chemotherapy if they had cancer due to the "devastating effects on the entire body and the immune system, and because of its extremely low success rate."[78]

Chemotherapy drugs are cytotoxic – toxic to living cells. This means that, although these drugs target fast-growing cancer cells to kill them, they also spread throughout the body killing other fast-growing cells such as those found in hair and the immune system. This is what accounts for chemotherapy's destructive side effects.[79] These side effects can include: bone marrow suppression, sore mouth, inflamed mucus membranes, nausea and vomiting, loss of appetite, changes in taste and smell, diarrhea, dehydration, constipation, fatigue, flu-like symptoms, hair loss, skin changes, eye changes, pain, cystitis, bedwetting, weight gain, pain at the injection site, inflamed vein, allergic reactions, fluid retention, organ damage, and secondary cancers.[80]

Chemotherapy drugs are poison and if given to healthy

77 *Cancer treatment and survivorship statistics*, 2012. Wiley Online Library. http://bit.ly/1gYDL2D

78 Wells, S D. *75% of physicians in the world refuse chemotherapy for themselves*. January 13, 2012. www.naturalnews.com/036054_chemotherapy_physicians_toxicity.html

79 Veracity, Dani. *Killer cancer treatment: How toxic chemotherapy kills both cancer cells and cancer patients*. October 25, 2005. http://bit.ly/1eJjn5F

80 *Side Effects of Chemotherapy*. Canadian Cancer Society. http://bit.ly/1t5kjL3

people, will make them very sick. So, what kind of reasoning is used to think it can be given to a sick person to poison them back to health? Chemotherapy does not address what is causing the cancer in the first place. It's like taking the battery out of your smoke alarm because it is making a noise, without looking for the source of the smoke and correcting that.

Chemotherapy causes a great deal of pain, suffering and fatigue, and seriously weakens the immune system, at least during treatment. After treatment, doctors use terms such as 'survival rate' and 'remission.' You are supposed to believe that if your cancer is in remission, it is cured. But this is a deception. The true definition of remission is only 'a reduction or absence of signs or symptoms.' Doctors can't find *evidence* of it on tests at that time. Another way of describing cancer going into remission is to say it has gone into hiding. Then, if and when it is strong enough to show itself again, it has usually spread – metastasized – to other parts of the body, and this time it comes back for the kill! What caused the cancer in the first place has not been dealt with.

The conventional cancer treatments of chemotherapy, radiation, and surgery treat only the *symptoms* of cancer. They do not address the cause of the cancer, which is a low level of oxygen in the affected cells. If the cause is not addressed and healed, the odds of the cancer returning are extremely high.

In Chapter 2, I told you that Otto Warburg discovered that cancer cannot grow when cellular oxygen levels are normal. I further explained that oxygen levels are normal when cellular fluids are near to the normal pH of 7. This happens when there is proper acid/alkaline balance in the body. So in a very real sense, we have come full circle in our discussion of health and disease. The best way to prevent disease, or work on treating it before it becomes serious, is to get back to the basics explained in this Disease-Free Revolution plan.

Cancer is a multi-billion dollar industry. Looking at it from a purely money-making and employment point of view, is it any wonder that people are led to believe that conventional treatments for cancer are the only or best solutions? Without an understanding about how and why cancer develops in the body, and lacking information regarding possible treatments or methods to reverse and correct the causes, people remain dependent on the treatments they are told about by their doctors. However, what we need to be asking is – do these treatments work to correct the cause of the cancer? There are other treatment alternatives; it just takes some work to find and understand them.

I hope that hearing about these health myths, or distortions of the facts, will encourage you to question other things we are told to accept as truths by the pharmaceutical, medical, and food industries. In order to be in control of your own health you need to become informed and make decisions that will help your body build the strong cells and immunity for you that it was designed to do. Remember that it is the questions you ask in life that are most important. Don't just accept things as fact before checking them out yourself just because some medical authority or media campaign tells you so. It may be true, but it may not be either. You need to check it out because it is your own health that is at stake.

In the next chapter I will present the how-to-do's and what-to-do's of building a healthy body. This is a tools-for-action chapter. Let's move on to consider some practical aspects of changing over to a healthier lifestyle and I encourage you to start putting them into action in your life right away. If we have knowledge but don't put it into practice, nothing changes. It is like a light switch that we never turn on. If you want the lights to come on in your life, you have to start switching on some of the healthy lifestyle practices.

CHAPTER 7

BUILDING A HEALTHY BODY
Part 1

In the chapters leading up to this one, I have tried to give you the background knowledge of how your body works and what it needs to be healthy. This Disease-Free Revolution program gives you the capability of using this knowledge to take the main responsibility for, and control of, your own health.

Although I could elaborate considerably on these and other subjects about natural health, the information here is distilled down to the basics and what is most important. I don't want you to feel overloaded or overwhelmed. Remember the basics and keep it as simple as possible. One natural health doctor I know says: "Clean and feed your body!" By that he means – consume foods, drinks, and supplements that will both clean your body of toxins and help it to build health.

I also like to put it another way: "Stop doing the wrong things and start doing the right things!" Take small steps at the beginning and keep moving forward. Read and re-read this Disease-Free Revolution program and use it as a reference as often as you need to. When you start on your healthy eating program but fall off a bit when you are eating out for example, don't beat yourself up about it. Just get back on the program and move ahead again. Tomorrow is another day. The important thing is to keep moving ahead with small steps of improvement.

In this chapter I will talk about:

- The true and very interesting story about the Pottenger Cats experiments and what we can learn from this study regarding our own health and disease processes
- Taking stock of your health situation as you start your health program
- How to monitor your own health by measuring your acid-alkaline balance at home
- Foods and drinks that should be avoided.

WHY YOU NEED TO TAKE CONTROL

I want to bring us back to the question: "Who is responsible for *your* health?" Other people might be sympathetic if you get sick or are suffering with a health condition, but it is you who is doing the suffering. It's your life. And to get out of that suffering or improve your situation you need to understand – nutritionally and natural-health-wise – how you got there. So I am going to tell you the true story about the Pottenger Cats, which illustrates the consequences of eating food that is not natural and does not contain enough live nutrition to create health in the long term.

The Pottenger cats study[81]

Dr. Francis Pottenger is one of my heroes. He was a medical doctor in California and he wanted to know the difference that eating raw versus cooked food makes to health. So from 1932 to 1942 he conducted nutritional experiments with 900 cats. He divided them into groups and fed them various combinations of raw and cooked food. But for simplicity sake we will talk about just two groups – the raw food cats and the cooked food cats. To maintain sperm consistency throughout the generations, all female cats were bred by raw-food males. Raw food cats were fed raw meat and raw unpasteurized milk. Cooked food cats were fed cooked meat and pasteurized milk. All cats were given a supplement of cod liver oil.

The results were as follows: the raw food cats continued to be healthy normal cats from generation to generation. However, cooking food can denature it in several ways making it a deficient diet for complete health. Mainly, enzymes are destroyed and protein is denatured which reduces or eliminates the ability of these proteins to be properly digested. As such, the first generation cooked-food cats developed diseases, illnesses, and deficiency symptoms –similar to what we see in our human population – near the end of their lives. Emotional and nervous problems began to appear. Structural problems in their bones and teeth began to happen. The second generation cooked-food cats developed disease problems around mid-life.

---

81   Pottenger, Francis M. Jr. MD. *Pottenger's Cats, A Study in Nutrition*. 2nd Edition. 1995. Price-Pottenger Nutrition Foundation, Inc. La Mesa CA. 91943-2614.

Third generation cooked-food cats developed disease problems at the beginning of their lives, with many dying before they were six months old. And here is the surprising part – there was no fourth generation cooked food cats produced! Either 3rd generation parents were sterile, or 4th generation cats were aborted before birth.

Some people might be saying: "Interesting, but we are not cats," and that's true. But while later studies have found that cooking food destroys *taurine*, which is an essential amino acid that cats must have to be healthy, cooking food also destroys another essential amino acid, *lysine,* which humans must have to be healthy. (The human body cannot manufacture lysine; it must be obtained from raw or partially-cooked food, such as nuts, beans, peas, lentils, meat, eggs, and raw-milk cheese.) Cooking at temperatures over 105 to 118 degrees Fahrenheit (40.5 to 48 degrees Celsius) also kills all the natural digestive enzymes in raw food. So in my opinion, we have much to take notice of from the Pottenger Cats experiment results.

Where is the good news?
The good news from the Pottenger Cats experiments is that when the cooked food cats were switched back to a healthy diet for cats, they gradually returned to normal health again. Depending on how many generations they had been on a deficient diet, it took from one to four generations to do this.

So, what about an eating plan for us?
Well, for us humans I am not suggesting that we must eat

an all-raw diet. I always suggest easing in to it gradually, with the eventual objective of achieving 50% raw. And even if you get partway there it will be a great improvement because millions of North Americans eat no raw food at all and very few vegetables.

Calories are misunderstood

Millions of people trying to lose weight are told to watch the amount of calories they eat because more calories tend to put on more weight. That is true – partly, because it is the calories and proteins in cooked food that are the problems. In recent studies, scientists have found that cooking food increases the amount of energy or calories that it provides to your body, whereas eating raw food leads to weight loss.[82] However, in my opinion, this is only part of the explanation. Cooking food may increase available calories but it also kills live nutrients such as enzymes and probiotics, and distorts protein molecules making them less bio-available to the human body. Further, because cooked protein molecules are changed from their natural configurations, the body sees them as foreign invaders and revs up the immune system to deal with them by increasing the white blood cell count.[83] This does not happen with raw foods because they retain all their live ingredients in a natural form that is easily recognized and processed by the body.

---

82   Arumugam, Nadia. *Eat Raw Food to Lose Weight, Cooked food Contains More Calories.* http://www.forbes.com/sites/nadiaarumugam/2011/12/28/eat-raw-food-to-lose-weight-cooked-food-contains-more-calories/

83   Dawn, Laura. *Cooked Protein vs. Raw Protein.* http://bit.ly/1m4FqeS

The body runs more efficiently with an adequate intake of raw food – both in digesting and metabolizing it, and in eliminating the wastes resulting from it. When one significantly increases the intake of raw organic ripe fruits and vegetables, the usual side benefit to feeling healthier is a shedding of some extra pounds of body weight. My conclusion regarding calories is that they certainly matter in cooked food, but have no consequence in a diet of raw food.

Introducing more raw food into your diet

If you are starting from a diet containing very little raw food, or if you are sick or elderly, you will need to take some time before you change over to more raw food. It is best to concentrate on nutritious soups and broths containing an assortment of cooked vegetables and some animal protein. As you gain in strength, add raw foods slowly to give your digestion system time to adjust to this new form of food.

A healthy diet takes time to transition to as you begin to feel the benefits of improved digestion, elimination, and more energy. It's not hard to do either when you are shown how. I like to say that changing over to the new healthier diet is an add-to diet, not a take-away diet. You gradually add more of the good foods to your plate and slowly reduce the not-so-good foods. In time, as your taste buds change their preferences, the good foods become more appealing and they tend to push some of the other foods off the plate. The slow and steady plan is best *unless* you are trying to correct a serious health situation and you don't have much time. In this case you would want to make the transition much faster.

How long does it take for changes to happen?

Since we live much longer than cats do, when we change over to a nutritious diet that satisfies our physical nutritional requirements and we work to detoxify our bodies, we can usually see improvements in energy and how we feel in a fairly short time. But if you already have a disease in progress, it could take several months to a few years to *completely* reverse the health damage that has been done in your body during your lifetime up until now. Like the cats, it depends on how serious our health conditions are when we start, and how serious we are in making the efforts and lifestyle changes that are needed. That part is up to you. How badly do you want it?

STARTING YOUR NEW HEALTH PROGRAM

As you start applying the Disease-Free Revolution health plan to your lifestyle it is a great idea to make a record of your present health situation. Write the date in a journal and list all the physical things that are bothering you at that time. Then each week, record your diet and lifestyle changes as well as your physical symptom changes as time goes along. If you have been doing what you need to do, I think you will be quite pleasantly surprised. Writing your symptoms down is important to give you the encouragement to carry on, because we naturally have a tendency to forget things that don't bother us anymore and then think that not much has changed. By doing this you will see that you are making progress and will be encouraged to continue.

Now let's get into the nuts and bolts of what to do and how to do it. We'll start by learning how to measure the state of your health and monitor your progress as you go along. In the second chapter I said that I would tell you later exactly how you can measure your body's acid-alkaline levels right in the privacy of your own home. By doing this you can check on your health progress. I believe that this is absolutely indispensable! When you are driving your car you need to see the road ahead of you. And to improve your health you need to know where your body chemistry is and where you want it to be. It is a roadmap that shows you what adjustments you need to make in your health-building program.

Remember that when your acid-alkaline levels are balanced your oxygen and energy levels are at their highest. Body cells and tissues then have a natural, strong immunity to all those bad bugs that like to set up shop inside us and start having lunch. Your body is in a strong state to be able to resist disease. This is the state we are aiming for. This is the condition that keeps disease away, moves you to your ideal weight, keeps you looking younger than your age and feeling good, and slows down the aging process in your body. The absolute highest and first priority in health is to balance your acid/alkaline levels. Without this, nothing works properly in your body.

In the second chapter I explained that we measure acid and alkaline strengths by using the pH scale. Readings increasing above 7.0 become more alkaline, and readings decreasing below 7.0 become more acidic. When pH is balanced at near-neutral, close to 7.0, that's when health is best. The important part to understand as far as health is concerned is that, as the pH of cellular and intra-cellular fluids becomes more acidic, this results in seriously lower levels of oxygen and energy production in cells. That's the territory in which the little disease bugs inside us take over and multiply.

Checking saliva and urine pH

The pH of saliva and urine when you first wake up are reliable indicators of the acidity or alkalinity of body fluids and tissues. Saliva pH indicates the strength of your body's alkaline reserve and therefore, your state of health; both are very closely related. The pH of the first urine in the morning shows you what your kidneys are filtering out of the blood to get rid of. Minerals that your body eliminates through urine are mainly the excess of either acid or alkaline water-soluble minerals. It gives you an indication of whether you fed your body an acidifying diet or an alkalizing diet. When alkaline mineral reserves have been exhausted the urine pH will always indicate acidity, except in cases of very serious illness when pH appears to be normal but actually is not. That is when the body is so acidic that, to save the kidneys from being burned by the strong acid coming into it with the blood, it produces its own strongly alkaline ammonia to weaken the acid. You may have smelled this odor in seniors' homes or in hospital palliative care wards for the terminally ill. This use of ammonia by the body is a survival mechanism in order to keep itself alive a little longer. You see, it always hopes that help will arrive in the form of detoxification and alkaline foods and supplements to help it return to health. It hangs on until the last possible moment.

In order to take readings of your saliva and urine pH you will need pH strips. These are usually available in health food stores. When you place a pH strip in your saliva or urine, the color of the strip changes to indicate the level of acidity or alkalinity of the fluid being measured. These pH strips are usually little paper rolls of litmus paper from which you can tear a piece to use each time. However, I sometimes find these papers hard to read in the way of getting an exact color. Also, if they have been on the shelf for too long they tend to become unreliable. I prefer to use 'pHydrion brilliant plastic dip sticks pH 5 to 9,' which can be bought online. They are reliable and very easy to read. I always keep some in my bathroom medicine cabinet.

Use a pH strip to check your saliva before getting out of bed or right away as soon as you get to the bathroom. Move your tongue a bit and swallow two or three times to get the saliva flowing and fresh. Touch the pH strip on your tongue to wet it, then remove it and take the reading by matching it against the color chart provided with the strips. Next, go to the bathroom to check the pH of your urine with another strip. You can quickly place the pH strip into the urine stream and remove it. Or you can urinate into a little cup or glass and then quickly dip the strip in and out again. Record both saliva and urine readings and keep track of them over time.

The ideal average first-in-the-morning reading for both saliva and urine is approximately 7.0. During the day both the saliva and urine readings will vary depending on what we eat and drink. Because our body filters out excess acids that are in the protein foods we eat, urine pH during the day will usually be lower. Ideal saliva pH readings should be: 6.8 when you wake up, 7.0 after getting up but before eating, and 8.5 after breakfast.

First-in-the-morning urine pH numbers are easier to understand. When body pH is in healthy balance, the urine has very little odor and has a pH in the range of 6.8 to 7.2. When urine pH is lower than 6.8, you have a clear indication that you need to increase your alkaline mineral reserves. To do this, eliminate as many of the acid-producing foods and beverages as possible and increase your intake of alkaline foods, drinks, and supplements. Lists of the main alkaline foods, acid foods, and drugs are listed in the appendices at the back of this book.

When a person is starting a switch-over health program from a less than ideal health position – meaning that the body is in an acidic state – the urine should always give an acidic reading because that is what the body is eliminating and replacing with alkaline minerals. As health improves the urine acidic readings will gradually move upward towards alkaline.

When body pH is very acidic

When first-in-the-morning urine pH readings are consistently acidic, that is below 6.1, this is an indication that your body is seriously deficient in alkaline minerals, especially organic sodium and potassium. These alkaline minerals *must* be replenished for true health to occur, because these acidic conditions are where all manner of disease conditions grow and multiply.

A stricter adherence to a diet of alkaline foods and beverages plus alkaline supplements if needed, and an avoidance of acid-producing foods is necessary to bring your body into a healthy acid-alkaline balance. Try to make these dietary changes gradually to allow your body time to adjust to new foods.

When all body systems are overly acidic, this indicates another seemingly contradictory problem. Although the body is overburdened with too much acid in its system, stomach acid, which is needed for digestion, is the body's first defence against pathogens entering the body with food, and is normally very strong with a pH between 1 and 3, becomes weaker. The stomach may not be producing *enough* acid to properly break down protein foods in digestion. The reason for this is that the stomach's hydrochloric acid-producing cells are so toxic they cannot work efficiently. In this case, supplementation with betaine hydrochloride and digestive enzymes before meals may be required as a temporary measure. The more acidic the body of the individual is, the more acid supplementation will be required to relieve their symptoms of digestive discomfort and improve digestion. These symptoms are often indigestion and heartburn, for which the standard remedy is antacids. Unfortunately, although this can give temporary relief, this is exactly the opposite of what is required because it does not address the *cause*, which is a *weak* presence of stomach acid. You can read more about this online under "why we need strong stomach acid."

My preference in these situations as a temporary measure is to use *unpasteurized* apple cider vinegar, which is rich in organic alkaline minerals. One teaspoonful or so can be taken in a little water before meals. This provides a remedial medium in the stomach and intestines that promotes digestion and assimilation of minerals. Unpasteurized apple cider vinegar is a live food which is acidic in the stomach, but which leaves an alkaline residue in the body after digestion.

Unprocessed sea salt is very useful as a source of organic sodium and many other minerals. One-half teaspoon or so of sea salt in a glass of water, right after getting up in the morning or as necessary, can be taken. Unprocessed sea salt is natural salt. Do not use table salt, sodium chloride, which is toxic and cannot be utilized by your body; it only contributes to a worsening of health problems. Kelp powder from pristine northern Atlantic waters is another good source of organic sodium and other minerals, including the very-important mineral iodine. Health suffers in many ways without adequate iodine.

Be patient and persistent

A body that is very acidic is lacking alkaline minerals and has probably been that way for many years. It can take several months of alkalizing and detoxification to fully correct a pH imbalance. Be patient but persistent during this process. Note that when one switches from unhealthy eating to healthy eating, and has started using alkaline foods and supplements, urine pH numbers can actually go down, becoming more acidic at first. Don't be alarmed because this is quite normal. As alkaline minerals are being supplied, your body will begin eliminating acid minerals from the areas it was previously forced to store them in. It will work to correct the most unhealthy acid terrain conditions immediately. In time, as alkaline minerals continue to be supplied in your food and mineral supplements, steady progress will be made as pH numbers move upward toward acid-alkaline balance.

As a personal example, before I started alkalizing I was getting urine pH readings in the 5.5 to 6 area. After I cut out the major acidifying foods and drinks and started alkalizing, my urine pH numbers went down to the 4.5 range which really frightened me *until* I studied carefully to understand what was going on. My body was dumping acidic minerals fast to get rid of them, and restoring its reserve of alkaline minerals. After my body had eliminated the stored acid minerals, my urine pH numbers steadily climbed toward 7.0.

Once acid-alkaline balance has been reached and has become stable, we can *occasionally* be less strict about what we eat. By monitoring our urine pH we can make diet and supplement corrections as needed to keep our cells producing optimum oxygen levels.

What to avoid

OK, now it's time to get into what we eat and drink. Let's start with the main ones we should avoid. Start by cutting out the worst and gradually work down the list. These are all acid-producing foods and many contain toxic chemicals that work against your body's efforts to build health. When you search for it you will find a long list of specific foods and beverages that should be avoided because they are acid-producing, but I don't want to overwhelm you or turn you off by listing them here. So instead, I will try to make general descriptions that will include most of them:

- Beverages and juices that contain alcohol, sugar, artificial sweeteners, table salt, preservatives, carbonation, or chemicals such as chlorine and fluoride in drinking water
- Anything containing caffeine, nicotine, sugar, or table salt
- Processed foods. Canned, packaged, or boxed foods, because almost all of them contain sugar, table salt, chemicals and preservatives. Don't believe me? Read the labels!
- Sugar in all its forms, except perhaps some natural unpasteurized honey in moderation
- All refined grains – most of the nutrition has been removed and the remaining refined carbohydrates are quickly converted to sugar in the body
- Fast foods – most contain sugar, table salt, and trans-fats
- All GMO – genetically modified foods
- Pasteurized dairy products
- The four bad whites – sugar, table salt, white rice, plus white flour and products made from it, which are white breads, pastas, cookies and pastries
- Egg substitutes
- Any meats from animals, birds, or fish, raised with hormones and/or antibiotics. (Pork is the least-healthy meat due to the variety of parasites in the meat that are difficult to kill even by cooking.)
- All foods fried in hot fats or oils

- Canned or frozen fruit concentrates – most are made from sub-standard produce which is acidic, and then more acid is added to give the products longer shelf life.

A little more detail on GMO foods

Genetically modified organisms (GMO) refer to plants or animals that have been genetically engineered (GE) to alter their DNA structure. GMO and GE foods are different words for the same thing. Using techniques of biotechnology, genes from one species are merged or inserted into the genes of another species to produce an organism whose DNA structure is different from that found in nature.

Gene splicing apparently dates back to 1972 and this technology entered the food system in 1990. It began in 1994 when Monsanto introduced a form of bovine growth hormone that was manufactured by genetically modified bacteria that farmers could inject into dairy cattle to increase milk production. The next step was to introduce genetically modified bacteria into the nucleus of plant cells. These techniques led to the development of Roundup-ready and other genetically modified crops.[84] Today, the list of genetically modified foods keeps getting longer and includes: corn, soy, tomatoes, dairy products, papayas, sugar, animal feed, salmon, golden rice, squash, sugar beets, potatoes, and oils such as canola.

GE seeds are developed to increase yields and to make plants resistant to insects, viruses, and herbicides. The herbicide Roundup, with its active ingredient glyphosate,

---

84   http://bit.ly/Rl7dLw

was developed by Monsanto and has been quickly adopted by farmers because of its ability to kill weeds without killing their crops, which has led to an increasing use of this herbicide. However in response, weeds are naturally adapting to these poisons and mutating to become 'superweeds,' which are Roundup-resistant. Also, this huge rise in glyphosate herbicide use is where health problems for us are developing.

A US study concluded that heavy use of the herbicide Roundup could be linked to a range of health problems and diseases. The study states that the negative impact of GE foods on the body is insidious and manifests slowly over time as inflammation damages cellular systems throughout the body.[85]

Dr. Dan Murphy, DC, in an article entitled *The Harmful Effects of GMO Foods,* said that glyphosate, the active ingredient in Roundup, may be the most biologically disruptive chemical in our environment. He further stated that exposure to this herbicide has been linked to liver and kidney dysfunction, greatly increased risk of cancer, shortened lifespan, inflammatory bowel diseases, Crohn's disease, chronic diarrhea, colitis, digestive issues, obesity, autism, Alzheimer's disease, depression, Parkinson's disease, leaky gut syndrome, multiple sclerosis, ADHD, violent impulsive behavior, suicide, infertility, preeclampsia, late-pregnancy spontaneous abortion, multiple myeloma, cardiovascular disease, cachexia, and ALS.[86]

---

85 http://reut.rs/1p5ZYph

86 Murphy, Dan. DC. *The Harmful Effects of GMO Foods.* The Specific Chiropractor Center. Draper. UT. http://on.fb.me/1jHcshM

However in spite of study conclusions, Monsanto and other chemical company scientists continue to argue that their products are safe and harmless. It reminds me of the tobacco company claims of fifty or so years ago that smoking was not harmful to health. I remember seeing ads of doctors smoking various brands of cigarettes – meant of course to assure us that smoking was OK. We now know the final outcome of those persuasions.

While the present standoff continues, not everyone is buying in to the chemical company arguments. Several European Union countries have banned the import of GMO crops, and a groundswell movement has begun in North America against GMO foods and demanding the labelling of foods containing genetically engineered ingredients.

Chemicals, preservatives, synthetic ingredients, and other additives in processed foods

The food we buy from stores, the cleaning fluids and cosmetics we use and the air we breathe are not what they used to be. One hundred years ago you could pretty well count on food being natural. That's not the case today. "There are more than 80,000 chemicals in the United States catalogued by government regulators, and the health risks of most of them are unknown."[87] These have found their way into our food, drinks, cosmetics, cleaning products, air, and almost everything in our everyday lives. Consequently, these unnatural chemicals are contributing

---

87   http://wapo.st/1kWc5U6

heavy toxic loads to our bodies which they must attempt to deal with.

Additives such as chemical flavor-enhancers, dyes, and preservatives in food products can cause or contribute to problems ranging from allergies to cancer. All synthetic additives are strong acid producers.

So, how can we start sorting out the good from the bad that we are putting into and on our bodies? We can start by…

READING THOSE LABELS

We need to become aware of the ingredients that are in the products we eat, put on our bodies, or clean with. To do this, we need to start reading labels!

If you are not already in this habit you may be in for a big surprise. For instance, most brands of toothpaste contain three ingredients that pose health risks if too much is swallowed. They include sorbitol, a sugar alcohol sweetener, which is a liquid that keeps toothpaste from drying out and acts as a laxative that can cause nausea, gas, diarrhea, and stomach cramps. Second is sodium lauryl sulphate, used in floor cleaners and engine degreasers. It is potentially carcinogenic and is a very strong irritant. Some toothpaste products contain TSP which is tri-sodium phosphate, a strong all-purpose cleaning chemical so strong it is used to clean grease off garage floors. It carries the general precaution: "Whenever handling TSP, be sure to wear rubber gloves or other protective material." And third, fluoride which displaces iodine in the body and is a poison if too much is swallowed. Some toothpaste labels contain a warning to get professional help, or call a poison control center immediately if someone has accidentally swallowed more than the amounts normally used for brushing teeth, which is described as a *pea-sized amount*. Do you use more than this? So when buying toothpaste, you should read the labels and choose an all-natural product.

Now I'm not just singling out toothpaste here. Almost all manufactured and processed products contain chemical additives and preservatives. Here is another example. Many underarm deodorants and antiperspirants contain aluminum, which is a toxic metal that has been associated with the development of dementia, Alzheimer's, and other diseases. While the function of these products is to close skin pores so that a person doesn't perspire or sweat in these areas, some of the chemicals in them are absorbed into their body where they become stored as toxic waste. If you do choose to use a deodorant, read the labels to ensure that it contains all-natural ingredients. And here's one thing to realize – when your body has become detoxified through your efforts and being on a good eating plan for a while, your perspiration will have very little odor to it anymore. The reason it does smell in the first place is because of a body that is so toxic it tries to sweat some of the poisons out through the skin to get rid of them. I don't use deodorants or antiperspirants anymore because I don't need them now that my body is clean inside and out.

The bottom line on processed food products, cleaning agents, or personal hygiene items that come in contact with our bodies is: if they aren't natural, your body cannot use them for health and they may even be outright harmful, if not in the short term, certainly in the long term.

Wherever you go to buy products at the grocery store, drug store, or health food store, the guideline for reading labels and selecting products is – as soon as you see an ingredient that is a chemical or a word that you can't pronounce, put it back! If you are still curious, make note of the questionable ingredient and search online to understand what it is. Your health depends on it and your body will thank you for it. There are always natural alternatives. You just may have to look for them. And don't just assume that all products in a health food store are pure and natural. You need to read *those* labels too.

In this chapter I have talked about why you need to be in control of your personal health program and how you can monitor your own state of health. Then I told you about the main foods and beverages you need to avoid because they are harmful to your health – if not in the short-term, certainly over the long-term.

In the next chapter, we will turn our attention to the good things – the food, drinks, and supplements you can use to build a healthy body with strong immunity. I will also give you a few easy suggestions and general eating rules to get you started on your new health program.

CHAPTER 8

BUILDING A HEALTHY BODY
Part 2

In this chapter I will talk about:

- Foods and drinks that build energy, health, and natural immunity
- Why buying organic foods is better
- The main supplements that can help on your road to vibrant health
- A few easy suggestions to get you started on your disease-free health plan
- General guidelines for healthy eating

Now let's get into the good things – the ones that really help your body be what you want it to be.

WATER

Our body is so dependent on water that without enough of it we would die in a few days. Approximately two-thirds of our body weight is water and our blood is about 90% water. Everything that happens in our body happens in a medium of water. It is our second most critical requirement after oxygen. Water is the main medium for transport of nutrients into tissues, and elimination of wastes from the body. It serves as the body's main lubricant and temperature regulator. Water is so critical to all body functions that even small decreases in body weight water bring on impairment of human performance, as indicated in the following chart:

Percent of Body Water Lost - Symptoms[88]

- 0% – none, optimal performance, normal heat regulation
- 1% – thirst stimulated, heat regulation during exercise altered, performance declines
- 2% – further decrease in heat regulation, hinders performance, increased thirst
- 3% – more of the same (worsening performance)
- 4% – exercise performance cut by 20 - 30%
- 5% – headache, irritability, "spaced-out" feeling, fatigue
- 6% – weakness, severe loss of thermoregulation
- 7% – collapse likely unless exercise stops
- 10% – comatose
- 11% – death likely

Even though we are often reminded to drink enough water to stay hydrated, it is estimated that over 80% of the American population suffers energy loss due to minor

88   Grandjean & Ruud. *Nutrition for Cyclists*, Clinics in Sports Med. Jan 1994. Vol. 13(1);235-246.

dehydration.[89] Clean water, and enough of it, is an absolute requirement for health. We need to get enough water from raw fruits and vegetables and from drinking good water every day. If we wait until we are feeling thirsty we are already starting to dehydrate.

Tap water is not always good

Many people do not realize that the water supplied in our city systems is not the best for their bodies. This is because it has been treated with chemicals such as chlorine and fluoride – both of which are harmful. At the very least, this water should be cleansed of chlorine by running it through a filtering unit in your kitchen. Removing fluoride from water is much more difficult. Alternatively, one can by bottled spring water.

Guidelines for drinking water

Raw fruits and vegetables naturally contain 75% to 90% water. They should be a major source of satisfying your body's requirement for water. Because of their high fiber content, these foods also contribute greatly to better elimination. They contain organic minerals your body needs and can easily use. The water in raw fruits and vegetables is pure, living water. On average, a person needs the equivalent of about 6 to 8 full glasses of clean water each day. Other liquids such as coffee, tea, soft drinks, and alcohol do not qualify as fluids that meet our daily water requirement because they cause your body extra work to process and eliminate them.

---

89   *The Health Benefits of Water*. www.dorchesterhealth.org/water.htm

Alcohol actually dehydrates all parts of the body.

From a good digestion point of view, water and other liquids should not be taken with meals because it dilutes digestive juices and interferes with digestion. Ice water does the same. Because it is so cold, it slows the digestive process down. Drinking distilled and reverse-osmosis water on a regular basis is not good either. These processes are used to make 'clean' water by boiling the water away from its minerals, or forcing water through an extremely fine membrane to remove dissolved minerals, respectively. The resulting water has an acidic pH, and over time it can contribute to nutritional imbalances in your body. These processes are different than running water through a tap or jug filtering unit which contain material to remove chlorine.

Generally, thirst should be our guide for drinking more water. Since water is of critical importance to life, these are some guidelines we should keep in mind for drinking water:

- Drink enough of it every day to satisfy your body's need for hydration
- Any kind of water is better than no water
- Water should be filtered to remove pollutants and chemicals, then re-mineralized with ionic minerals or a little sea salt or even fresh-squeezed lemon juice. Juice from ripe raw lemons leaves an alkaline residue in the body after digestion.
- Slightly alkaline water from a spring or artesian well is best. Some bottled waters are available from these sources.

Those are the basics you need to know about water.

DIGESTIVE ENZYMES

As I briefly mentioned in Chapter 2, digestive enzymes are a natural part of all living foods – living catalysts that activate all biochemical reactions in our bodies; they make things happen. Along with probiotics or friendly bacteria in your colon, enzymes are the workers in your body. It is only when food is processed that these enzymes are killed, causing your body to use its own precious stored nutritional resources to manufacture them itself to help with digestion. It can do this but it takes a steady toll on your vitality and brings on age-related problems earlier.

There are basically two kinds of enzymes: digestive enzymes, which are supplied from raw, living food; and metabolic enzymes that your body manufactures for cell growth and to keep your tissues and organs maintained. We only need to be concerned with digestive enzymes in our health programs because the metabolic enzymes are made in your body automatically.

The main digestive enzymes are a combination of:

- Amylase – to digest carbohydrates, such as bread, pasta, potatoes, white rice, etc.
- Protease – to digest proteins, such as meat, fish, beans, protein powders, etc.
- Lipase – to digest fats and oils
- Cellulase – needed to break down the fibers in fruits and vegetables.

There are two ways to get digestive enzymes. The first is from raw food we eat. The second is from supplements that we can buy. Digestive enzymes should always contain a combination of at least the above four enzymes, and they usually also include other enzymes to help break down sugars and lactose from milk, for example. On a program to regain one's health, it is a great help to your body to take two or three digestive enzyme capsules every time you eat cooked food.

MINERALS

Most people know that we need proteins and carbohydrates from our food, but we seem to take minerals for granted or don't realize how important they are. Minerals are the sparkplugs of life in your body. They are the foundation of your electrical system and the catalysts for hundreds of metabolic enzyme reactions within your body. Without a reasonable supply and balance of minerals your body slips into disease. We cannot manufacture minerals in our body; they must be obtained from the food we eat. Lack of minerals is a major contributor to health problems today. The best source of minerals is from a variety of fruits and vegetables and natural sea salt, which contains about 84 minerals and trace minerals.

Why buying organic produce is better

Most of our fruit, grain, and vegetable foods are now grown in soils that have been depleted of minerals due to over-farming. Soils have also been treated with pesticides and chemical fertilizers. Fruit and vegetables are picked before they are ripe and have not had time to gather all their nutrients. Most produce that is shipped across state and country borders has been radiated, which kills enzymes. What we end up with is food that is nutrient-deficient, bland-tasting, and not suitable to build complete health. The taste comparison between commercially-grown produce and that which has been grown in a home garden, fertilized with organic compost or animal manure, is quite evident. It only makes common sense that soil, which is continually farmed and fertilized with only three or four chemicals each year, will become depleted of its minerals and trace elements. Vegetables can be grown in this manner that look good, but they lack their full compliment of minerals because each year fewer trace minerals are left in the soil.

The best solution to the problem of nutrient-deficient food is to buy organic food from local small farms as much as possible, because certified organic farming is done without the use of pesticides or chemical fertilizers. Organic farm soils are enriched naturally with compost materials and animal fertilizers that contain a variety of organic nutrients and living organisms which create healthy soil. Tests have proven that the mineral content of organic produce is superior to most commercially-farmed produce. Of course, organizations that have vested interests in promoting produce grown on over-farmed soils with chemical fertilizers come up with their own studies to refute this. However, one particularly well-researched book called *The Healing Power of Minerals, Special Nutrients and Trace Elements* by Paul Bergner is very convincing. It includes figures that show a decline in mineral content of several fruits and vegetables over a 30-year period.

Average changes in the mineral content of some fruits and vegetables, 1963-1992.[90]

Mineral	Average % Change
Calcium	-29.82
Iron	-32.00
Magnesium	-21.08
Phosphorus	-11.09
Potassium	-6.48

Without a steady supply of alkaline minerals, such as calcium, magnesium, and potassium, the human body slips into acidosis and it's just a matter of time before disease begins to develop. That's why I recommend you try to spend the extra money to buy organic food which can feed your body now, rather than buying produce that leads to mineral deficiencies and disease in your body, and consequently higher medical bills, later. When you pay a little more to buy organic, just look at it as buying good health insurance.

If you are able to buy only the standard commercial produce, try to also use a good, natural mineral supplement plus digestive enzymes with meals as well. It is also best to thoroughly wash the produce before eating to remove as many pesticides as possible.

Don't be fooled by the word 'natural' on labels. There can be a big difference between 'natural' and 'organic.'

---

90 Diver, Steve. *Nutritional Quality of Organically Grown Food*. 2002. http://bit.ly/1hEo1GU

By law and third-party certification, organic food and organic food products must be produced without the use of synthetic pesticides and chemical fertilizers, drugs given to animals, genetically modified organisms (GMOs), irradiation, nanoparticles, or sewage sludge fertilizers. On the other hand, products called 'natural' are completely unregulated. You don't know what is in them or what processing was used to arrive at the final product. So to be safe, always buy certified organic whenever you can.

A caution for those who are sick now, and those who have weak digestive systems

While raw food contains all the living nutrition necessary to build life and should usually make up 50% of a healthy diet, in times of illness it may not be the best for your body. The reason is that raw food, with the exception of freshly-made low-sweet fruit and vegetable juices, takes too much energy to digest when a person is sick and the nutrition may just pass through them. This is when we need to turn to home-made soups, broths, and lightly steamed and cooked foods, supplemented with digestive enzymes. Raw vegetables, especially starchy ones, have the minerals locked in their fibers. A weak digestive system lacks the energy to break these down so it can use the nutrients from the fibers. Cooking does this. If sick people and people with weak digestive systems continue with a mostly raw-food diet for too long, they run the risk of eventually demineralizing their bodies. So the advice here is to first begin to build up mineral reserves with soups, broths, and lightly steamed vegetables (no more than 8 minutes recommended for most), eaten with supplemental digestive enzymes. As energy and health return, raw foods can again be slowly introduced, especially in the form of freshly-made low-sweet fruit and vegetable juices and smoothies, which I will talk about next.

JUICING

Making and consuming fresh, raw, low-sweet fruit and vegetable juices regularly can be one of the fastest ways of returning to vibrant health. The reasons for this are that freshly-made juices take very little energy for digestion – only about 10% of that required by solid food. You can heal in one month of juicing what would take you six months on good solid food.[91] Fresh juices made from organic fruits and vegetables are alkaline and chock-full of vital nutrients that your body can put to use quickly. An extra bonus is that they really help your body to detoxify and restore its alkaline mineral reserves. When juicing, always try to use organic produce because it has more minerals and is free of pesticide toxins. I suggest that you use mostly vegetables such as carrot, celery, kale, spinach, and a small amount of beet or ginger root.

Try your own combinations, but keep in mind that organic kale and carrot are usually the foundation vegetables for juicing. The one caution I have, and it is a strong one, is to go easy on fruits, especially sweet fruits. Although they taste very good, many of them are loaded with the simple sugar fructose, and without fiber from the whole fruit, they quickly raise the level of sugar in your bloodstream. We

91 Dr. Joel Robbins, DC, ND, MD. College of Natural Health. Tulsa, OK.

don't want that because sugar causes inflammation in the body. Fructose can also cause problems in the liver leading to an increase in body fat plus insulin resistance and Type II diabetes.

Smoothies

Smoothies are like freshly-made juices, except the fiber is left in. They are made using a high-speed blender. Smoothies are easy to make with any combination of fruit and vegetables. High-speed blenders have the ability to break down the cellulose fibres in raw fruits and vegetables to release their nutrition, and that is something that our bodies can have difficulty doing on their own. This kind of blending can greatly increase the percentage of nutrients available for digestion and assimilation.

Green vegetable smoothies are one of the most nutritious meals one can eat, especially when made with organic ingredients. They are tasty and quick to prepare.

An ordinary blender can be used, but a high-speed blender is more powerful and efficient. The basic green smoothie instructions for one person are: blend a handful of greens, such as spinach, kale, romaine lettuce, and/or parsley, with two glasses of water. Then add a ripe banana or apple, and one or two tablespoons of a low-heat processed protein powder (such as rice or whey protein). Blend the mix until it is creamy. You can vary the recipe each day according to your taste, flavouring it with mint, dill, lemon juice, or whatever you find appealing. When changing your eating plan a smoothie can be an excellent easy-to-make lunch meal. You can also make it in the morning to take to work with you. It will lose some of its live qualities over a few hours but it still provides nutrition far superior to sandwiches or typical restaurant food.

SUPPLEMENTS

One of the first health books I read was, *Food is Your Best Medicine* by Dr. Henry Bieler. It contained the truth about where our main nutrition should come from, and that is whole foods. However, when our body systems are weakened and tired, or when we are fighting a disease condition, and when our foods don't have the full range of vitamins and minerals they should have, food supplements can play a vital and very helpful role.

I believe that the most important supplements to add to your eating plan include: digestive enzymes, probiotics (the good bowel bacteria), a good bowel-cleansing and rebuilding product, such as Herb Cocktail, a low-heat processed vegetable protein powder, chlorella and spirulina, and vitamin D3. Other good ones are krill oil or cod liver oil for their Omega 3 fatty acids, and North Sea kelp powder for its full range of sea minerals including iodine, which almost all North Americans are deficient in.

Guidelines for taking supplements

Supplements can play an important role in paying back deficiency debts to the body created by years of consuming nutrient-deficient food. True supplements are composed of whole food ingredients; they feed the body with balanced nutrients it can use to heal itself. It is my belief that when the body has been starved of vital nutrients or has been abused from an intake of improper nutrition and toxic substances, supplements are needed to correct deficiencies.

Many people take supplements of one form or another in attempts to ensure they are getting what may be deficient in the food they eat. The business of supplements is a huge, multi-billion dollar industry. Recent surveys show that 68% of Americans[92] and 33% of people in the UK[93] take nutritional supplements. However, not all supplements supply the life forces the body needs to regenerate itself. Many vitamins sold in drugstores and even in healthfood stores are chemically derived, synthetic, and therefore do not contain the organic components required by the body to build health. In fact, they may actually contribute to vitamin and mineral imbalances.

Because there are so many different kinds of supplements available, the decisions of what to believe and what to take have become confusing. In some ways it is like the prescription and over-the-counter drugs markets.

The truth is that certain supplements can be good and even necessary. The reason for nutritional supplements has developed because much of our modern-day food is nutritionally deficient due to over-farming and use of chemical fertilizers. This can lead to vitamin and mineral deficiencies in our bodies. There are facts you should know so that you can choose wisely when it comes to supplementing your diet with nutritional capsules or pills. Notice that the supplement recommendations I made in

92 http://bit.ly/1iRNs3T

93 http://bit.ly/1txFO7q

the previous section were quite simple. Here are a few important considerations when choosing supplements.

Supplements:

- Are meant to supplement the diet, not replace it or cause imbalances in the body
- Should be natural, not synthetic
- Should be manufactured using low-heat processes, as usually indicated on the label
- Should retain their life forces, and be made from combinations of various foods
- Should not be single minerals, because these cause imbalances. All natural foods contain minerals in combination with other elements
- Should be food-based as found in nature, with their vitamin and mineral co-factors intact
- Should not be in high doses, which can cause stimulation and imbalances in the body. With high doses, the body is stimulated to get rid of the excess which can deplete energy reserves and cause other deficiencies.

In my opinion, your main source for nutrition should always be from organically-raised produce – whole foods. However, good supplements can help make up for non-organic foods that are mineral deficient. Just be sure to choose supplements that are as close to nature as possible because these supplements can help your body heal, instead of giving it more stress and problems to deal with, as can be the case with chemical and synthetic supplements.

Testing for mineral deficiencies

In the previous section I talked about mineral deficiencies in the body that are caused by inadequate nutrition. But how can we tell if we are deficient in certain minerals in order to take sensible corrective action with foods and supplements? It is not a good idea to just take a shotgun approach and begin taking a lot of vitamins and minerals because we could be making matters worse for the body.

From my experience and knowledge, the only accurate way to determine one's mineral levels is to have a hair tissue mineral analysis done.[94] However, this is a very specialized science. According to Dr. L Wilson, there are very few health practitioners and laboratories that really understand how to do this testing properly and are able to interpret results correctly. Dr. Wilson has more than 30 years experience in nutritional balancing based on analysis of hair samples. He has continued with his development of this science and works with health practitioners throughout the world who are trained to follow his protocols.[95]

Healthy food practices

As we have discussed, we should aim for an eventual 50% raw in our eating plan with an alkaline to acid mix of about 80% alkaline to 20% acidic foods.

---

94   Wilson, Lawrence. MD. *Nutritional Balancing, An Introduction.* The Center for Development. 2012. www.drlwilson.com/articles/NUT.%20 BAL%20INTRO.htm

95   Wilson, Lawrence. MD. *Find a Nutritional Balancing Practitioner.* 2014. http://drlwilson.com/do%20hair%20analysis.htm

Healthy food practices include:

- Eat raw vegetables, non-sweet fruits, nuts, and seeds. Nuts and seeds soaked overnight are best, because this activates their natural enzymes and softens fibers for easier digestion

- When choosing meat, chicken, or fish, try to buy organic – free of hormones and antibiotics. This is becoming more and more important because of the alarming increase of antibiotic-resistant 'super germs' that have now evolved due to the overuse of antibiotics in both medicine and agriculture. To reduce your risk of encountering these super germs, avoid taking antibiotics unless absolutely necessary and avoid consuming meats containing antibiotics. Also avoid eating farm-raised fish, no matter what country they come from. I eat organic meat once every two or three weeks. The main advantage of eating a little red meat is that it contains the most abundant source of Iron and Vitamin B12, which your body needs to make healthy blood and energy

- Avoid food from cans or packages because it comes with the health–depleting additives of sugar, table salt, and hundreds of different chemicals. Also, chemicals leach into foods from the cans themselves and from plastics that have been heated in a microwave oven

- Shop for locally-grown, whole organic foods as much as possible. Go to farmers' markets and talk to the growers about how they grow the produce and how they raise the meat animals

- Avoid genetically modified foods like the plague. Our

bodies are not designed to use GMO foods

- Use digestive enzymes when eating cooked, processed, or irradiated foods. Digestive enzymes can also be taken on an empty stomach to help your body clean and rebuild itself

- Make detoxification a regular practice with the foods you eat by extending the time in the morning before eating cooked food, and not eating in the evening after dinner.

HEALTHY LIFESTYLE PRACTICE

- Do moderate exercise such as walking for 30 minutes each day, plus a few minutes of stretching and other mild exercises. A few minutes of light to moderate weight-bearing exercises are also helpful to maintain muscle mass. Your whole body depends on exercise for healthy blood circulation, movement of cellular wastes through the lymph system, and to generate electrical energy with your muscles.

Get enough sleep each night.

Remember that your body can only heal properly when at rest. Also, the energy we enjoy during the day was made while our body was asleep the previous night. If we don't get adequate sleep, these important functions cannot be accomplished efficiently. But as your health improves and the more detoxified your body becomes, the less sleep it will require. Most adults need at least eight hours of sleep each night, although this varies from person to person. So try to figure out how much sleep you need to feel at your best the next day.

Some tips for getting a good night's sleep:

- Go to bed at a regular time each night
- Take a nap during the day if you need to, and are able to do it, to catch up
- Make your bedroom as dark as possible to increase melatonin production by your pineal gland. Melatonin is a natural hormone produced by your body, primarily in darkness, to tell your brain when it is time to sleep
- Have your bedroom quiet and cool
- Don't turn on the light when you go to the bathroom during the night because this will break the melatonin cycle. Use a small flashlight if you need to
- Don't watch TV while you are in bed
- Avoid eating and drinking in the evening
- Try relaxation techniques if you need them, such as deep breathing, progressive muscle relaxing, and visualizing peaceful scenes.

A FEW EASY AND HELPFUL THINGS TO START ON

- First, as soon as you get up in the morning drink two glasses of filtered, room-temperature or warm water with the juice of one-half a fresh lemon squeezed into it. Or you can add one or two teaspoonfuls of unpasteurized apple cider vinegar to the water
- Second, try not to eat cooked food for as long as you can in the morning to extend your body's natural detoxification cycle
- Third, use digestive enzymes with cooked food
- Fourth, make green smoothies for lunch or snacks. These provide great nutrition and are an excellent source of fiber.

The general rules for eating are:

- Eat only real foods that are natural for your body – made by nature! No junk food or food from cans or packages
- Stop eating when you feel yourself getting full
- Reduce the amount of meat you eat
- Avoid refined sugar in all its forms, and sugar substitutes. Use natural sweeteners such as unpasteurized honey and maple syrup in moderation
- Avoid table salt. Use unprocessed sea salt
- Drink clean, filtered water
- Increase vegetables and non-sweet fruits in your diet
- Incorporate green smoothies into your diet

When you stay with this eating plan, the easier it will get and the more health benefits you will enjoy. If you fall off your eating plan occasionally, don't feel bad. Just get back with the program the next day. Help your body to detoxify from the meal or party the evening before by moving to healthy liquids – lots of good water with fresh lemon juice or unpasteurized apple cider vinegar, fresh vegetable juices, and diluted smoothies.

DO YOU WANT TO LOSE WEIGHT QUICKLY

When you follow the guidelines of The Disease-Free Revolution health plan, you will gradually lose weight – *if you need to* – at the same time you are rebuilding your health. However, some people might want to speed up their weight loss program, and there is a way to do it while still giving your body the nutrition it needs to be healthy, now and for the long term. Are you ready for something different?

In the sixth chapter I explained why most bodies put on weight and stay that way. The main reason a person puts on extra fat is due to eating a diet of almost all processed foods and acidic beverages. Their body's organs and channels of elimination become congested – plugged up! When a body cannot get rid of nutrition-less calories, wastes, and harmful toxins, it must store them as fat.

Let me tell you a true story. A woman friend of mine in her early fifties had not been feeling as well as she used to. She was tired and felt listless and unmotivated most of the time. She wanted to change something and feel healthier. Losing weight was not on her mind at the time. But she decided to eat an all raw-food diet for a while. She found a good raw food recipe book and started on her program. Very soon she started to notice some changes. Her bowel movements improved and became regular. Her energy came back and she felt more motivated and alive. She slept more restfully. As time went on her skin started to look better. Then after two months she noticed that her clothes were loose and she had lost 20 pounds. This was a bonus she had not expected. When I saw her with a group of friends just after her two months on raw food, everyone complimented her on how good she looked.

The reason for the good results is totally in line with The Disease-Free Revolution eating plan. When her body was getting live, active foods, it was able to easily digest and assimilate them. She was getting lots of natural digestive enzymes and alkaline minerals. Her organs of elimination started moving and detoxifying her body. One thing she said to me was that for a while, she was always hungry and had to keep eating. The reason for this sudden hunger needs to be understood.

Since her body had been starved for good nutrition for so long, as soon as the totally useable food started coming in, her body was constantly eliminating stored toxins and storing up good nutrition. As the toxins went out so did the fat they had been stored in. Her body was rebuilding as quickly as it was able to. When I saw her she looked healthy and said that she felt great. I don't think there is any need to say more. That example tells it all.

Eating a diet of raw low-sweet fruits and vegetables for a while can be easy when you make different kinds of smoothies an important part of your diet. They are quick and easy to make and taste great when you get the ingredients to your liking.

HEALTH IS LOST OR WON IN THE GUT

What you are about to read in this section is life-changing because it explains the basic cause of most of the disease conditions our society suffers from. The majority of this information is sourced from Douglas Wyatt, founder of the Center for Nutritional Research, and from the book, *Peptide Immunotherapy: A Physician's Guide,* by Dr. Andrew Keech.

In medical terminology, the word 'gut' refers to the intestines. In Chapter 2, I commented that many health practitioners use the phrase 'disease begins in the colon.' This is true because when rotting and stagnant fecal matter becomes congested in the colon, toxins are formed which begin to congest and reduce the efficiency of other organs. But that is only part of the story. What is not widely recognized, and is overlooked by many medical practitioners, is what happens upstream from the colon in the small intestine. Hippocrates, who lived in ancient Greece and is recognized as the father of western medicine, stated that, "All disease begins in the gut."

The problem

Influenced by poor lifestyle choices, the small intestine can develop tiny holes or perforations in its mucus lining, thereby becoming leaky. The small intestine is not supposed to have these perforations. However, when they do develop, the gut's protective walls become weak, which allows incompletely-digested proteins, fats, toxins, and bacteria to leak through into the blood stream, causing inflammation in various areas of the body. This condition is called Leaky Gut Syndrome and it is the basis for chronic disease. It is estimated that at least half the adult population and many children in the United States have Leaky Gut Syndrome.

A situation similar to leaky gut occurs with allergies. Allergens are able to enter and cause problems in the body due to weakened membranes of the skin, nose, sinus, throat, lungs, or intestines. Irritation and inflammation cause microscopic holes to develop and although very small, they are large enough to allow protein particles from pollen, animal dander, food, or other contaminants to gain entrance into the bloodstream. Acting in the interest of survival, the body's immune system works to eliminate these foreign substances. This results in inflammation, mucus discharge, itching, irritability, and reduced immune function.

Inflammation is present in most disease conditions. As an immune system response to irritation or damage, inflammation is the initial phase of the body's healing. When intestinal inflammation and leaky gut become chronic, healthy areas of the body become susceptible to damage as well. Leaky gut can be a problem for people of all ages. It can be the root cause of many health disorders and autoimmune conditions ranging from: indigestion, bowel disorders, malabsorption and deficiency of nutrients, chronic fatigue, memory problems, allergies, Candida, and skin problems such as eczema, to asthma, diabetes, cardiovascular conditions, Alzheimer's disease, autism, fibromyalgia, Crohn's disease, HIV/AIDS, multiple sclerosis, lupus, cancer, and numerous other autoimmune disorders.

The main causes of leaky gut include: overuse of antibiotics, meats containing antibiotics, over-the-counter and prescription pain medications, steroids, gastro-intestinal drugs, birth control pills, pesticide-laden foods, mold, Candida yeast overgrowth, bacteria, excessive ingestion of wheat products, GMO foods, sugar, caffeine, alcohol, some food additives, and chronic stress. Adults who were not breast-fed as babies also have a compromised gut system which originated in infancy.

Allergies and autoimmune disorders

Allergies and autoimmune diseases are almost always associated with Leaky Gut Syndrome.

The connection between Leaky Gut Syndrome and (many) autoimmune conditions is that the antibodies created by the body, in response to the toxic substances and undigested fats and proteins that leak into the bloodstream and attach themselves to various tissues throughout the body, create an allergic response, trigger destruction of tissues and organs, and create inflammation.[96]

In the case of allergies, the immune system becomes hypersensitive and reacts to an outside substance that it would normally ignore. With autoimmune conditions, the immune system reacts to normal body tissues and begins attacking them as if they were foreign invaders; it produces antibodies against its own tissues. Under the conditions of increasing toxicity and chronic inflammation in the gut, the immune system becomes overactive and confused and can no longer tell the difference between healthy body tissues and antigens; it produces a response that destroys healthy normal tissue.

The specific type of autoimmune disease that develops depends on the predominant location of the inflammation.[97]

Since the gut immune system contains 70 to 80% of the body's immune cells,[98] it is obvious that this is the area of our body that needs assistance if we wish to improve our health.

---

96   Wyatt, Douglas. *A. Leaky Gut Syndrome: A Modern Epidemic with an Ancient Solution?* Center for Nutritional Research.

97   Ibid.

98   Furness, John. B., Kunze, Wolfgang. A. A., Clerc, Nadine. *The intestine as a sensory organ: neural, endocrine, and immune responses.* American Journal of Physiology - Gastrointestinal and Liver Physiology Published 1 November 1999Vol. 277no. G922-G928. http://ajpgi.physiology.org/content/277/5/G922

The solution – bioactive colostrum

It seems that any time we stray too far from Mother Nature's way of caring for our bodies we run into difficulties. Altered foods, chemical drugs, preservatives, and pollutants are not natural to the human body and sooner or later they force body systems out of balance. It should be no surprise to us that nature had the prescription to being healthy from the beginning of our lives, and nature also offers the possible solution to correct health problems as we grow older.

When mammals are born, their first food is colostrum from their mothers. This first milk, or actually 'pre-milk,' is very special because it transfers the all-important immune and growth factors plus nutrients from mother to infant.

The newborn gut is unique in that it has not completed maturation at the time of birth and needs the growth factors and other components of the mother's colostrum to complete its development. This incomplete development of the gut is of benefit to the newborn as it allows large proteins, such as immunoglobulins, to easily enter the body. Immunoglobulins in colostrum and mother's milk bind to disease-causing pathogens on the mucosal surfaces of the GI tract, thereby preventing them from colonizing and causing infection. This modulation by the immune system creates passive immunity for the infant.[99]

Shortly after ingesting immune-strengthening colostrum, the porous openings in the infant's gut close to provide a protective barrier so that large protein particles from

99   Wyatt, Douglas. A. *Bovine Colostrum and Post-Pregnancy Re-vitalization.* Vital Health News. www.centerfornutritionalresearch.org

food, plus viruses and bacteria cannot enter directly into the bloodstream. This protective barrier remains intact until one or more of the factors mentioned above cause the small intestine to become injured and porous. Fortunately for us, when we consume colostrum it can provide the same healing benefits and immune fortification that infants who are breast-fed this first food receive. Not only can colostrum heal holes in the gut, but it can also repair mucus lining perforations throughout the rest of the body that cause allergic reactions.

Of course as adults we do not consume colostrum from human mother's milk, but there is a wonderful alternative. Colostrum produced by cows – bovine colostrum – is bi-oidentical to human colostrum, yet it contains significantly higher levels of the immunoglobulin IgG, which can neutralize microorganisms, many of which are now resistant to present-day antibiotics. It contains powerful antibacterial and antiviral factors. Therefore, as an immune enhancement, bovine colostrum is even better than human colostrum.

Bovine colostrum contains hundreds of thousands of components, of which only a few hundred have been identified and studied, that enhance the human body's functioning by two primary mechanisms. First, the numerous immune factors and natural antibiotics in colostrum provide strong support for optimal immune system performance. Second, colostrum's growth factors offer a broad-spectrum boost for optimal health and tissue healing.[100]

---

100 Wyatt, Douglas. A. *Anti-Aging Benefits of Bovine Colostrum*. Vital Health News. www.centerfornutritionalresearch.org

The gland in our bodies responsible for producing T cells, which are major components of the body's immune response to foreign invaders and infections, is the thymus. The thymus gland is located behind the sternum in our chest just in front of the heart. This gland grows to the approximate size of an orange until we reach puberty, and then begins to shrink. By the time we are 70 years old, the thymus gland has reduced to approximately the size of a pea. This is one explanation of why we have weaker immune systems as we age. Bovine colostrum is able to restore the thymus gland to optimal functioning capacity and correct an underactive immune system. According to Doug Wyatt, who has been working with physicians for over two decades, people who have been supplementing with bovine colostrum consistently and over time, report that they do not get colds or the flu anymore. And, people who start taking colostrum when they are already sick with a viral or bacterial infection report greatly accelerated healing and recovery times.

Dr. Donald Henderson, MD, and Professor of Medicine at UCLA, stated:

> Colostrum is the ideal solution for Leaky Gut Syndrome. Its components prevent and heal GI damage. Unless the gut is healed, the body cannot begin the process of repair.

Benefits of consuming colostrum

Bovine colostrum is not a medicine or a drug; it is a superfood that is whole and natural. It is able to stimulate an underactive immune system or modulate an overactive one.

It is also able to increase growth hormones in the body to restore a more youthful functioning of many physiological processes and promote growth of body tissues. Thousands of clinical trials have proven colostrum to be safe and effective, with no known drug interactions or adverse side effects. It is the perfect food to assist in the recovery from all disease conditions.

Researchers have found that nutrients in colostrum are directly responsible for the production of stem cells in our bone marrow. "When they measured the before and after stem cell counts in the blood, virtually none are detected prior. Within a week of consuming, trillions of stem cells can be found." Nothing other than colostrum has been clinically proven to stimulate the production of stem cells.[101]

The only food that was designed to heal, protect, and make our gastro-intestinal tract perfect is colostrum. When this first pre-milk food, containing high levels of its active components, is regularly consumed and the leaky gut situation is healed, many health benefits can start to be realized. Some of the main ones include: improved digestion and bowel function, increased energy and feelings of well-being, faster healing after injuries, repair of DNA and RNA, regulated blood sugar levels, increased infection control, improved memory, building of lean muscle and bone density, increased endurance, reduction of body fat, more youthful skin appearance, and improved sexual function.

---

101 Wyatt, Douglas. The Key to Health and Longevity: Colostrum.
http://www.sovereignlaboratories.com/info_KEYTOHEALTH.html

Active bovine colostrum has been referred to as the closest thing we have to a fountain of youth. As we age, it can give us a renewed lease on life.

Anti-aging

After we are born, the thymus gland, which produces the major components for our body's immune response system, reaches maximum size and function at puberty and then continues to atrophy as we grow older. As it shrinks, the production of T-cell immunity factors reduces accordingly,[102] and the incidence of age-related diseases increases.[103] A similar pattern occurs with the body's growth factors.

Growth hormone (GH), often referred to as human growth hormone (HGH), is produced by the pituitary gland in the brain. Levels of growth hormones continue to be high during the early stage of life to promote tissue and bone growth until adult size and reproductive maturation are attained. After this, GH production in the body decreases steadily as we age, to the point that a 60 year old may secrete only 25% of that secreted by a 20 year old.[104] Some symptoms that can accompany GH decline include: reduced muscle size and strength, weight gain – especially around the abdomen, low energy, weight loss,

102 Whitman, Deborah. B. *The Immunology of Aging*. March 1999. http://www.csa.com/discoveryguides/archives/immune-aging.php

103 Kelley, Keith. W. Professor of Immunophysiology, Department of Animal Sciences, University of Illinois. *Biotechnology of Aging*. http://www.aces.uiuc.edu/vista/html_pubs/irspsm91/aging.html

104 Anti-Aging and Wellness Center. *Human Growth Hormone* (HGH). http://www.antiagingwellnesscenter.com/hgh.shtml

mood swings, poorer memory, thinner skin, wrinkles, greying and falling hair, slower healing of wounds, sleep difficulties, and diminished libido.

In recent years there has been much publicity regarding the advantages of taking HGH injections or HGH precursors, which stimulate the pituitary gland to produce more growth hormone. They can act in a similar manner to drugs. Results have shown that various anti-aging benefits can be achieved by doing this. However, in my opinion there is a problem with this approach because the delicate balance of hormones, as well as natural hormone production in the body, can be very easily upset. This is similar to imbalance problems that can be created by taking isolated vitamins and minerals. Our bodies were made to be nourished by natural whole foods that provide complete, not isolated, nutritional factors. This is where colostrum can provide a natural solution to slow and even reverse some of the undesirable effects of aging.

Bovine colostrum is a totally natural, complete, and balanced food. It is rich in the youth-promoting insulin-like growth factors IGF-1 and IGF-2, which have regenerative effects that extend to nearly all structural cells of the body. Bovine colostrum promotes healing and anti-aging effects by returning body growth factors to pre-puberty levels, with the results of increasing muscle mass and strength as well as stimulating growth and repair of DNA and RNA.[105]

A study with older adults found that supplementing

105 Wyatt, Douglas. *Anti-Aging Benefits of Bovine Colostrum.* colostrumtherapy.com

with colostrum can be beneficial for enhancing muscular strength – up to 20% increase in lower body strength – and preventing bone loss. The study noted that this is significant because older adults lose muscle mass and strength in the lower body more quickly than in the upper body.[106]

Colostrum improves athletic performance

Bovine colostrum is not just for those with health problems, because healthy people can enjoy significant benefits from it as well. Clinical studies of athletes supplementing with bovine colostrum have shown impressive results including up to 20% more lean muscle strength, increased stamina and performance, less susceptibiity to after-workout infections, accelerated healing from injuries and strenuous physical exertion, plus enhanced brain chemical response for better visualizations and concentration.[107]

The right kind of colostrum

Not all colostrum products are the same, nor are they equally effective. As mentioned in the last paragraph, a colostrum product must contain high levels of its original active components in order to bring about healing. Colostrum's effectiveness depends on its source and how it has been processed. Consequently, health results can vary widely based on the quality of the colostrum you consume.

Good colostrum comes from healthy cows that are

---

106 The Colostrum Counsel – *Bovine Colostrum Supplementing Exercise in the Older Adult*. www.saskatooncolostrum.com

107 Wyatt, Doug. Colostrum LD: *Truly A Miracle Food*. www.sovereignlaboratories.com

pasture-fed and raised without antibiotics or hormones. It must not be processed under high heat because this destroys much of its biological activity. It must not have been frozen either. The final colostrum product should be water-soluble so it can disperse well in the gut. In its original form fresh from the cow, colostrum particles are coated with a lipid (oil) layer so they can survive the stomach's harsh environment and arrive in the small intestine intact to deliver their health-giving components. Therefore, the processing of colostrum for long-term storage must also include a treatment that coats its particles with a protective lipid so it can function with the same effectiveness as fresh colostrum. See Appendix 3 for a source that meets all the above criteria.

> If your colostrum is heat-dried, not end product tested for bioactivity and does not have the LD (Liposomal Delivery) reapplied to the dried colostrum, it is no more effective than powdered milk. – *Andrew Keech, PhD*

Final comment regarding bovine colostrum and leaky gut
Bovine colostrum does not cure any disease on its own – only the body can do that when it has a balanced immune system and the required nutritional factors. What colostrum can do is heal a leaky gut and other porous mucus membranes. In addition, it can provide powerful immune-strengthening and anti-aging benefits with its immunoglobulin, growth, and nutritional factors. If all this sounds too good to be true, it is not – because this is what nature intended and created colostrum to do. This is its function.

This is very exciting information for correcting a

weakened immune system and the many health problems related to it. You cannot enjoy a disease-free life without having a healthy intestinal tract and a strong immune system. My advice is to give bovine colostrum a try. You may be very pleasantly surprised by the results of supplementing with it. Just be sure of the source and quality of the product when you buy colostrum.

WHEN YOU NEED FURTHER INFORMATION

Sometimes, even when you have a pretty firm understanding of the natural health principles explained in this teaching series, questions can come up in your mind when you are experiencing some minor health problem and you might want further information. When this happens to me I go online, because there is a wealth of information of all kinds to be found there. The main problem is to know *how* to search for it. My suggestion is to type into a search engine such as Google on the Internet, the problem or issue you want to know more about. Then also type in the words 'natural' or 'natural cure' or 'natural approach.' By doing this you will find more natural health suggestions and not be focussed only on medical sites, which are often associated with pharmaceutical or surgical solutions. Also, be sure to type in the word 'cause' so you can work on actually correcting the situation you are concerned about, and not be just addressing symptoms.

Learning is all about asking questions and knowing *how* to search for the information you want. That's what we were supposed to have been taught in school

– how to be independent thinkers and *how* to learn new information – not to just accept what we were told. Your independence and freedom in all areas of your life depend on you questioning things you are told to accept – before accepting them! It also depends on your ability and desire to search for new information, and then use it in your thinking process to decide what action or solution is in your own best interests. This is a very important part of taking responsibility for your own health and life, *and* of being successful.

PHARMACEUTICAL DRUGS AND VACCINATIONS

While drugs may be necessary to combat some infections and can save lives under serious or traumatic circumstances, they are not natural to the human body and cannot *build* health or correct bodily nutritional deficiencies. They are chemicals, lacking life themselves. I'll repeat that – drugs can save lives and relieve symptoms of disease such as pain, but they cannot build health. In many cases their continued use works against long-term health. If they have to be used I think they should be used only as a temporary measure. Always be thinking about how you can work with your body using natural methods.

You may be interested to know that the use of pharmaceuticals by the medical system is barely one hundred years old. Drugs were not mandated as the only approved treatment by the medical profession until the very early 1900s. Prior to this time, all medical schools in America taught the use of only natural remedies for healing. However, this was competition that the pharmaceutical interests of the day were determined to organize against and legislate out of the way.[108]

I ask you to think about the possibility that the drug and vaccination industries may not always have your best interests in mind. They may be more concerned about making money than they are about making you healthy. At the beginning of the 1900s, Sir William Osler, who lived from 1849 to 1919 and was one of the four founding professors at Johns Hopkins Hospital in Baltimore Maryland, stated:

> Drug companies are not here to bring us health, but to scam us for vast amounts of money, by treating symptoms and not addressing the cause.[109]

I encourage you to use your own wisdom and discernment regarding all matters concerning your health and your life. If you don't exercise your own right to direct your own life, someone else will always be ready to take control for you.

CANCER

I am often asked what a person can do about cancer because, as I mentioned in the sixth chapter, fear is often used by medical authorities to promote the treatment modes of chemotherapy, radiation, or surgery. And make no mistake about it; a diagnosis of cancer is very scary.

---

108 Robbins, Joel, DC, ND, MD. *Health Through Nutrition.* 1992. pp. 55, 56.

109 http://blueprintwellnessinc.com/

But the low success rates of these conventional cancer treatments are also very scary and not encouraging. And with chemotherapy, there are so many unpleasant side affects. As a friend of mine said a few years after he had undergone chemotherapy treatments for cancer, and when the cancer symptoms were starting to return again: "After chemo, your quality of life is never the same."

From my experience, I believe that the degree of health and immune system strength of every person are different and therefore, each case of cancer is different. The more you study and learn about cancer, the more you will understand that other treatment modes are available. You just have to find out about them because medical doctors are not allowed to tell you about them – even if they might know about them. You won't learn about alternative treatments from the medical or pharmaceutical industry practitioners. However, naturopathic doctors may be a source for non-pharmaceutical approaches to treating cancer. They are also more likely to advise you about your body's nutritional requirements during and after treatment.

To my knowledge, the best place to start finding alternative treatments for cancer is to go to the website cancertutor. com. There is lots of wonderful information there. A great book on cancer is: *Cancer – Step Outside the Box,* by Ty Bollinger. Dr. L. Wilson, MD, also has an excellent article entitled *Cancer and Alternative Therapies.*[110] You just have to sort through all this the information and make your own decisions. Start reading, studying, and making notes as you

---

110 http://drlwilson.com/articles/CANCER%20INT.htm

search for alternative approaches that work on correcting the *causes* of your own specific health challenges. In the meantime, the most important thing you can do is work to improve the health of your digestive tract and the strength of your immune system, and to my knowledge, the best food supplement for this is bovine colostrum.

In my opinion, the main points to keep in mind regarding cancer are:

- Dr. Otto Warburg discovered that cancer occurs whenever any cell is denied 60% of its oxygen requirements
- Cells with an acidic pH have low levels of oxygen
- Cancer cannot survive and grow when cellular oxygen is normal
- Oxygen is normal when cellular pH is slightly alkaline
- If cellular pH can be raised to alkaline, oxygen is increased and cancer cells die
- Cancer cells surround themselves with a protective fibrin coating to avoid recognition by the body's immune system[111]. This coating is difficult to break through. The rest of the body cells can be alkaline but being protected, the cancer cells can still continue growing
- It appears that the key to killing cancer cells is to find elements and nutritional components that can enter the affected cells to raise the internal pH so that oxygen levels return to normal.

---

111 Lipinski, B; Egyud, L. G. *Resistance of cancer cells to immune recognition and killing.* Abstract 2000 Mar:54 (3) 456-60. PubMed.gov. http://www.ncbi. nlm.nih.gov/pubmed/10783488

When this kind of approach is taken to treating cancer, one is attempting to address the cause of the cancer and not be simply focussed on removing the symptoms. Of course, at the same time, one must be working to detoxify and nourish the body with wholesome foods and beverages such as you have learned about in this book.

THE RADIATION THREAT

Over the past several decades the world has been increasingly subjected to the health threats of radiation poisoning. Exposure to bursts of high level or continuing low levels of radiation is proven to cause cancer. Nuclear radiation is also known as ionizing radiation, which means that it has the ability to change the electron structure of atoms that are exposed to it. In human and animal tissue these changes result in damage to DNA, the carrier of genetic information within cells. If this damage is not repaired by the body, it can lead to many types of cancer in the years following exposure.

Where is radiation exposure to the general public coming from? First it was the atmospheric nuclear bomb testing of the 1940s, 50s, and 60s. Then it was the development of nuclear reactors for generation of electricity. As of December 31, 2012, there were 437 nuclear power plants in operation around the world.[112] This is where the main radiation threats to our health are coming from. The Chernobyl disaster occurred on April 26, 1986. Deaths

---

112 Nuclear Technology Review 2013. p. 5. http://www.iaea.org/About/
     Policy/GC/GC57/GC57InfDocuments/English/gc57inf-2_en.pdf

between 1986 and 2004 resulting from this accident are estimated to be 985,000 – mostly from cancers, with more deaths projected to follow.[113] Most recent was the meltdown of nuclear reactors in Fukushima, Japan which occurred in 2011 as a result of an earthquake and a tidal wave that swamped the power plants. Serious radioactivity was, and still is being released into the atmosphere and the Pacific Ocean. And, of course, because air and ocean currents circulate around the world, the effects of this radiation are affecting everyone to a greater or lesser degree.

The big question regarding the radioactive threat is, "Do we need to fear it?" If we do nothing to protect ourselves, the answer is probably – yes. But we should be aware of it and we need to respect its potential for harm so that we can take steps to reduce our fears and protect our health. A very inspiring video produced by Markus Rothkranz entitled: *Don't Fear Radiation,*[114] recently came to my attention. It features interviews with two people who survived high nuclear radiation exposure and are now thriving. The first is Katrine Volynsky of Russia, who recovered from the Chernobyl disaster and now teaches people how to be healthy in an unhealthy world. The second person interviewed is US nuclear test pilot Captain Gary Pylant, now 70, who survived exposure to nuclear blasts, and actually flew his plane through a highly radioactive mushroom cloud created from an atomic bomb

113 Grossman, Carl. *Chernobyl Death Toll 985,000, Mostly From Cancer.* March 13, 2013. http://forums.canadiancontent.net/technology/114688-chernobyl-death-toll-985-000-a.html

114 http://bit.ly/1kW9DNs (February 13, 2014)

test in Nevada. All of his fellow pilots and crew on these assignments have since died.

What are the survival and health secrets of these two amazing people? Well, as it turns out, they are not secrets at all – just known and practiced by very few people. They are the same powerful health principles you are learning about in this book, *The Disease-Free Revolution*. In short, they are: regular detoxification with emphasis on keeping the colon and liver clean with fiber, colonics, and coffee-retention enemas; French green clay to remove radiation and heavy metals; whole organic foods, including lots of fresh raw green juices and smoothies; re-mineralizing the body; exercise; and, a positive "I can do it" attitude. What these two individuals are doing – and you can too – is harnessing the powerful survival desire, instinct, and reparative capability of the human body, by cooperating with it and giving it the tools it needs to combat disease and regenerate health.

PREVENTION OF DISEASE IS ALWAYS BEST

Remember the old saying that: "An ounce of prevention is worth a pound of cure!" It's a lot less painful too.

Hopefully, you do not yet have what might be considered to be a terminal illness and you can change the acidic and toxic problems in your body before a serious disease does start to show itself. And even if you do suffer from a disease condition, then the first and highest priorities are alkaline nutrition and detoxification. However, your best solution to avoiding disease is always prevention. That's why I wrote this *Disease-Free Revolution* book. My strongest recommendation is for you to put these health principles into practice in your own life and start right now on the road to being disease-free and enjoying your right to health freedom.

THE MAIN KEY TO A LONG LIFE

Most of this book is devoted to showing you how to keep your internal organs clean, and how to choose food that will nourish your body so you can be toxin-free as much as possible to live a disease-free life. This means that you need to be conscious of your diet and lifestyle practices and be persistent with your good habits – you have to be conscientious about it.

The Longevity Project[115] is the title of a book that reports the results of an extensive study of 1500 bright American children beginning in 1921 and following them through life, interviewing them repeatedly over eight decades. The intent of this project was to attempt to identify which traits contribute to a long life, and why? Of course, many were identified but there was one overriding factor. The conclusion may surprise you, but considering what I said in the paragraph before this one, it may not. The main factor predictive of longevity is a personality trait – conscientiousness! When we think about it, this is logical because conscientious people are dependable, hardworking, persistent, and well-organized. They are more likely to take care of their health, eat healthy foods, engage in fewer risky

---

115 Friedman, Howard S. PhD, and Martin, Leslie R. *The Longevity Project*. Plume Publishing. 2012.

behaviors, be more involved in healthy social activities, help others, and have good friendships.[116]

This is encouraging and reinforcing. Conscientious people tend to be happier than those who are not. They are usually busy and occupied with activities. They stay active and involved with others. They make their lives interesting and enjoyable because their first priority is to take care of their own health so they will have the energy and feelings of well-being to stay active.

If you want to live a long life full of health and happiness, the message is clear – be conscientious about putting your health first. Good examples of this can be found in the health transformation stories in Appendix 1 at the end of this book. Make a health plan for yourself and stick to it. When you feel truly healthy, all the rest that life has to offer can follow. Then you can really enjoy your long life and be an inspiration and a helping friend to others.

YOU CAN DO IT

As I end this book I would like to wish you all the very best in your search for lasting good health. I'm confident it is there – if you are willing to go for it. I leave you with a challenge. That challenge is to create a vision of health for yourself. Decide exactly what you want to achieve in your health program. Write it down on paper along with the date. Call it: "My vision for my health." Then list and describe the things you want to change and improve. That

---

116 Selig, Meg. What is the Essential Key to a Long Life? Psychology Today. March 23, 2011. http://bit.ly/1gyCwb6

is, write down all the health symptoms that are bothering you.

Set goals and small steps for yourself – detoxification goals; gradual, better nutrition goals; how you will add nutritious foods, eliminate bad foods, drinks, and habits; moderate exercise goals such as walking and stretching; how you are going to work on your attitudes and beliefs to remove any painful blockages from the past, including forgiving others and especially yourself. Make a calendar of dates for when you will do a one day vegetable juice fast, then maybe a two or three-day vegetable juice or watermelon fast. Then do them. Your body will love you for it. Remember – small steps. Then as time goes by, keep adding more. Your health program is about progress, not perfection. You don't have to be perfect to be good. Focus on what you can do, where you are, with what you have, and those little changes will add up.

This is *your* program and *your* decision. Don't expect all your friends and family members to be as enthusiastic about it as you are. Let them do what they want to do and you follow your own eating and detoxification programs *quietly* and with determination. Family members are often among the hardest to convince. Don't be a preacher about your new health program. Just get on it and keep moving ahead. In time, as your health starts to change for the better, others will begin to take notice and comment or ask what you are doing. If they are really interested for themselves, you will then have the knowledge and experience to help them. That's what I have done and I sincerely hope it gives you the inspiration and motivation to make the changes you would like to see in *your* life.

You now have health knowledge that very few people have – even many health practitioners. I believe it is information that should be taught in our schools. It is a gift of health knowledge that I hope you will use. Remember that knowledge is power, but *only* if you take action with it. And for almost everybody – *health* is a *choice,* when you know *what* to do, and *you do it.*

I've done my part. Now the rest is up to you as you join thousands of others in the disease-free revolution. Let's make a real difference in the world as we work to be examples of health and vitality well into our senior years.

Good luck as you start your new health program

This health plan is a program of freedom – freedom to be in control, and freedom from disease. For the great majority of people health is a choice – *when* you have the knowledge, and *when* you follow through with action. Yours can be a life of empowerment and hope.

If you are suffering from a disease right now, there is always hope for health. No matter what disease condition you may have, as long as your body has life and a little energy, and there have not been too many medical, surgical, chemical, or radiation interventions, it knows how to get well. Your body is capable of healing but it needs your full cooperation.

The human body is a wonderful creation. And because it has built-in intelligence, it is the best doctor in the world. It doesn't make mistakes. We do. Everything it does, it does on purpose. It always works to survive another day and become healthier, but it needs our help to supply good nutrition, assistance with detoxification, moderate exercise, and proper mental attitudes. There are many cases of people who have recovered from so-called 'death sentence' diseases.

To *everyone* I say again, *congratulations* for wanting to learn about how to take control of your own health program. If you don't want to be one of the disease statistics I talked about in the earlier chapters, this Disease-Free Revolution plan gives you the knowledge you need to change that for yourself. You *can* have a life of health, happiness, more energy, and joy. You have been given the plan, now the rest is up to you.

Hang in there and keep trying. Stay with your Disease-Free Revolution program. Make it your lifestyle.

APPENDIX 1

HEALTH TRANSFORMATION STORIES

The Disease-Free Revolution is a new and updated version of my earlier books which received enthusiastic reviews from readers and from those who changed their lives by following the health principles taught in them. Here are a few stories:

1. Hagen Von Conruhds, 82, was suffering with Lou Gehrig's disease (ALS). He drove many miles one evening on short notice to meet with me at a speaking engagement I had in his area. He told me that he had read one of my earlier books six times, and after strictly following the health principles in it, he had astounded his doctors in Vancouver, BC, Canada, by walking in to their office for a previously scheduled medical examination. Evidently, his earlier condition had been degrading so quickly that they expected him to be wheelchair-bound by that time, and they had not even been prepared for the examination. Hagen has survived with ALS for 12 years as of this date. This is quite remarkable, considering that only ten percent of people with this disease live more than ten years.

2. Lynne Garner, 71, a family member, had been on medications for many years for a neurological disorder that weakens muscles. She totally believed in the conventional medical system. But by age 70 her problems worsened to the point that she had put on a lot of weight and fluid, and was very exhausted. If she got down to tie her shoes, she couldn't get up by herself. She had to use a wheelchair when she went out. She could no longer drive her car. Her brain fog became so bad that it was difficult for her to organize her thoughts or make decisions. Her son, who was familiar with the health principles in my book, phoned me practically in tears one day, saying he was literally watching his mother die before his eyes, and was there anything he could do? His mother was resisting anything not conventional medical. After our discussion he asked his mother to try the natural health principles in my book. He challenged her by saying – "What have you got to lose?" Within a short time the weight started to come off and her energy began to return. A few months later, she was again walking stairs and managing on her own. Then she drove her car on a return trip of over 800 miles to visit a friend. She is still working on it, gradually reducing her medications, and continuing to make health gains.

3. Wanetta Beal, 41, is a personal fitness trainer in Coombs, BC, Canada.
"My road to health has been a journey. At age 24, I was a size 20, suffered from depression, bipolar disorder, severe irritable bowel syndrome, and was told I would be on several medications for life. The long-term side effects of these medications were potentially worse than the symptoms they were supposed to help. I was sick and tired of being sick and tired. I began losing weight and

went on to become a personal fitness trainer. I was slimmer but still on medications and still suffering. It wasn't until I read Ron Garner's book and began applying the health principles explained in it that my health really started to change. Within six months I was off all my medications, including Lithium, and my irritable bowel was a thing of the past.

My health has continued to improve and I have lost 76 pounds. I have been able to challenge my body way beyond what is considered normal. I have cycled to Alaska, Mexico, and across Canada. I ran the West Coast Trail on Vancouver Island – a rugged 75 kilometres, in one day. I ran the length of Vancouver Island, 498 kilometres, in nine consecutive days. I became the first woman to complete three Ironman Triathlons in 70 hours. Previously, no woman had completed more than one. I feel that I am able to do these things because of what I learned from Ron's book. My husband and I own a fitness gym where we share this information. Ron's book is one book we insist that all of our clients read. The results we have seen with our clients have been nothing short of miraculous. His book is a life-saver … literally!"

4. Lisalotte Meyer, 65, was overweight and had diabetes. She spoke at a health conference I attended in Red Deer, Alberta, Canada where she told the audience that after following the principles in my book she completely turned her health around. She lost 45 pounds and cured her diabetes – confirmed by her medical doctor.

5. Mandy Dugas, 28. British Columbia, Canada.

"I grew up on a meat and potatoes diet, and in my 20s lived on pizza, fast food, micro-waved, processed, and packaged food. I drank liquor, smoked, was overweight and always too tired to exercise. I was plagued with numerous allergies and throat infections. To make matters worse, my young son developed eczema all over his body and was often sick. I did exactly what the doctor told me to do but repeated visits to the hospital and antibiotic treatments did not stop his illnesses. I was envious of the vitality and energy that runners had and I wondered why my son and I couldn't have that kind of health. I was very unhappy.

I met my husband Tod, in 2011. He had a healthy glow that attracted me to him. He was a runner and I wanted to be healthy like him. I asked him how he did it and he said he followed the advice in a book called Conscious Health by Ron Garner. As I began reading this book I was sceptical because it went against my lifestyle and everything I had been brainwashed to believe. However, it had worked for Tod so I changed my diet and lifestyle and, as I followed Ron's recommendations I began to feel awesome. I changed my son's diet too and after a while his eczema started to fade and we both were rarely sick. I lost weight, my skin cleared, my monthly cycle cramps disappeared and I finally had the energy and desire to start exercising.

When Tod and I married in 2012 we tried to have a baby, but without success. I emailed Ron asking him for help. He suggested a couple of dietary changes which I made right away – and I got pregnant that month! The pregnancy went very smoothly and I exercised until 8.5 months.

We now have a beautiful healthy baby girl. She had one minor cold in her first year and has had no teething pain. She has clear skin, bright eyes, and is a perfect example of health because she has had the benefit of Ron's nutritional knowledge from day one.

I am happy and excited about my life now. We owe all our thanks to Ron and his books. They are life-changers, and we recommend them to our family and friends when they remark on our glowing health and want to know how we did it. Thank you Ron!"

GOOD FOOD AND LIFESTYLE PRACTICES SUMMARY

Reversing degenerative disease conditions and regaining good health can be accomplished more quickly by doing those things that have a very high impact on your body's ability to heal. It's really quite simple. Stop doing the wrong things and start doing the right things. Then keep doing them. Here is a brief list of the main healthy routines to put into your program:

- Eliminate all harmful foods from your diet
- Once each month fast for one or two days on fresh low-sweet fruit and vegetable juices, or eat only organic watermelon. Watermelon is easy to digest and satisfies the urge to chew
- Drink enough slightly alkaline water to satisfy body needs. Spring and artesian well water are best
- Use unpasteurized apple cider vinegar
- Drink freshly-made raw low-sweet fruit and vegetable juices regularly
- Make and consume a green smoothie every day
- Eat sprouted seeds – alfalfa, chick peas, mung beans
- Eat only when hungry
- Do not eat or drink after the dinner meal. This leaves 12 to 16 hours for your body to naturally process nutrition and detoxify until the morning meal when you 'break

the fast.' Doing this provides a huge assist to your body

- Eat 20% less at each meal for more efficient digestion and fewer calories
- Eat 80% alkaline, 20% acid-forming foods. If you are not in good health right now, make as close to 100% alkaline choices as you can until your acid-alkaline levels improve
- Gradually work up to eating 50% raw and 50% cooked food
- Moderately use only cheese made from unpasteurized (raw) milk
- If you are sick, weak, or elderly, eat more cooked foods with emphasis on home-made soups and broths
- Combine foods properly – eat fruits alone, and don't mix proteins with carbohydrates and sugars
- Eat plain yogurt, kefir, and fermented vegetables to increase probiotics in your digestive system. Goat milk and plain goat yogurt are better for your body than products made from cow's milk
- Eat organic eggs from free-run chickens; these eggs are a complete food
- Supplement with digestive enzymes, probiotics (bowel bacteria), and good oils
- Get 8 or 9 hours of sleep each night. This is when your body makes new energy and when it heals. If you constantly go short of sleep, your body cannot win the health game for you
- Walk every day. Even 15 to 30 minutes brings good rewards
- Adopt positive thoughts and attitudes

- Reduce stress in your life
- Work to keep your colon clean and bowel movements regular.

Superfoods

You already know about the kinds of food you need to concentrate on to feed your body what it needs to be healthy. Here are a few special health-building foods:

- Bovine colostrum – contains powerful immune, growth, anti-aging, nutritional, and healing factors. Also very helpful for gastro-intestinal and bowel disorders
- Bee pollen and royal jelly
- Unpasteurized apple cider vinegar
- Whole-leaf Aloe Vera juice – great for healing the entire intestinal tract
- Klamath Lake algae
- Organic coconut oil
- Raw goji berries
- Raw chocolate, called cacao. It contains no sugar
- Hemp foods – seeds, oil, and protein
- Fish oil and krill oil
- Vitamin D.

When you stay with the *Disease-Free Revolution* eating plan, it will get easier and you will begin to enjoy more health benefits as you go along, and you can move to a healthy weight that is natural for your body.

HEALTH PRODUCTS I USE OR CONSIDER TO BE GOOD

Note: These are my opinions only. I have no financial interest in the businesses or products listed below, with the exception of Avena Originals networking company of which I am a member because I believe these supplements are high-quality and most of all – they work for me.

1. Food
- All food should be certified organic. Meat, poultry, and fish should be raised without hormones or antibiotics.
- Buy local as much as possible.

2. Supplements
- Digestive enzymes, Probiotics, Vegetable-source protein powder (for smoothies), Superfood capsules of powder (greens and herbs) – Can be found in most health food stores. I buy mine from avenaoriginals.com
- Vitamins and Minerals - Can be found in most health food stores.
- Bovine Colostrum - soverignlaboratories.com
- Eye health - EYEMAX-*plus* Vision and Body Formula. Cambridge Institute for Better Vision. bettervision.com. (It is my opinion that this supplement is controlling and improving the macular degeneration I have as a genetic factor in my family.)

3. Detoxification

- Colon cleansing. Many products are available from health food stores. I use Herb Cocktail from avenaoriginals.com and consider it to be the foundation product of my health program.

4. Blenders for Making Smoothies

- There are several high-speed blenders available online. If you can afford it, try to buy one that has a motor rating of between 2 HP and 3.5 HP. These blenders are fairly expensive, but are very powerful, efficient, and easy to clean. They break down food fibers to release the minerals inside, and liquefy fruits and vegetables. I have owned one of these units for 17 years and use it every day.

5. Juicers

- There are many juicers available online. Look for one with a wide feed chute and sufficient power.

6. Measuring Acid-Alkaline Balance – pH strips

- Usually available from health food stores (ask to make sure the strips are not old). These are OK but can sometimes be hard to determine exact color
- Hydrion (9400) Spectral 5.0-9.0 Plastic pH Strips. These are easy to read and last a long time. They are available online.

APPENDIX 4

ALKALINE-FORMING AND ACID-FORMING FOODS

Many foods of one type, as they pass through our bodies, are acted upon by the body chemistry so that they produce an acid or alkaline residue (ash) that is the opposite of their original chemical composition. That is, some foods that are acidic, will alkalize, and vice versa. The following foods are listed in order, from most alkaline to most acidic; or, in other words, from most healthy to most harmful for the body.[117]

ALKALINE-FORMING[118]

- Raw fruits and their fresh juices
- Dried fruits
- Raw vegetables and their fresh juices
- Herbal teas
- Frozen fruits and vegetables
- Lightly steamed fruits and vegetables
- Raw nuts (almonds, pecans, et cetera)
- Raw seeds (sesame, pumpkin, squash, sunflower, et cetera)
- Sprouted grains

117 Robbins, Joel, DC, ND, MD, *Health Through Nutrition*. 1992. p. 15.

118 Baroody, Theodore A., ND, DC, PhD. *Alkalize or Die*. 2002.

ACID-FORMING

- Some raw fruits and vegetables (cranberries, plums, prunes, squash)
- Whole grains—cooked
- Overcooked fruits and vegetables
- Dairy products (cheese, milk)
- Eggs
- Sugar and refined grains
- Spices (dried mustard, nutmeg)
- White meats (fish, fowl)
- Fried foods
- Coffee and tea
- Red meats (beef, lamb, pork)
- Refined salt
- Soft drinks
- Alcohol
- Drugs and medications
- Tobacco

Note: A healthy diet should consist of approximately 70-80% alkaline foods and 20-30% acid foods.

ALKALINE FOODS

MODERATE TO STRONG ALKALINE

Raw fruits: Highest – melons, lemons, grapefruit, limes, mango, papaya, bananas

Raw vegetables: Highest – asparagus, carrots, celery, parsley, sea weed – kelp, algae

Beans: Green, lima

Herbs/Spices: Chives, garlic, vegetable salt, cayenne, unpasteurized apple cider vinegar

Grains: Arrowroot flour, Essene (manna) bread.
(All grains are alkaline when sprouted)

Protein: Bee pollen, royal jelly, milk from almonds and hempseeds

Nuts (moderate): Almonds, fresh coconut

Seeds: Most sprouted seeds

Sugars: Unpasteurized honey, stevia

Beverages: Fresh fruit and vegetable juices, herbal teas – alfalfa, clover, mint, sage

Digestive enzymes, green vegetable drinks, chlorophyll

Minerals: Sodium, potassium calcium, magnesium,

MILDLY ALKALINE

Raw fruits: Oranges, cherries, tart apples, Cucumbers, tomatoes, zucchini, bell peppers
Raw vegetables: Beets, cabbage, cauliflower, corn, kale, leeks, mushrooms, onions, peppers, radishes, potatoes with peel
Beans: Other beans, peas, string
Herbs/Spices: Most herbs and spices, Sea Salt
Grains: Amaranth, millet, quinoa
Protein: Vegetable proteins
Natural cottage cheese, yogurt
Oils: Most cold-pressed, fresh, untreated oils are neutral to slightly alkaline-forming
Beverages: Herbal teas – Strawberry, raspberry, ginger, comfrey, ginseng

ACIDIC FOODS

MILDLY ACIDIC

Fruits: Blueberries, cranberries, plums, prunes
Vegetables: Corn, lentils, olives, winter squash
Grains: Barley, rye, spelt, corn meal, buckwheat
Unrefined cereals, crackers, Popcorn – plain, butter (unsalted)
Proteins: Unpasteurized dairy, eggs
All raw nuts (except raw almonds and fresh coconut)
Seeds: Most unsprouted seeds
Sugars: Maple sugar, pasteurized honey, molasses, fructose, turbinado

MODERATE TO STRONGLY ACIDIC

Fruits: Green or over-ripe fruit
Most fast food products
Table salt
White vinegar
Grains: Rice and wheat (esp. white), oats, pancakes, waffles, muffins
Refined breads, pastas, pastries, cereals, crackers
Proteins: All meat, fish, fowl
Processed dairy, ice cream
All roasted and salted nuts

Oils: Avoid all heated, hydrogenated
Seeds: All roasted and salted seeds
Sugars: White processed sugar, artificial sweeteners
Beverages: Coffee and substitutes, black tea
All liquor: beer, wine
Soft drinks, carbonated drinks

All drugs, tobacco

ALKALIZING BROTH

One of the least expensive, yet very effective ways of improving your health and raising your pH to less acidic is to consume mineral-rich vegetable broth. This can be easily made at home using alkaline vegetables and a good vegetable salt. The broth will be rich in potassium, calcium, magnesium and sodium. Four or five cups of broth can be consumed each day that one is on a detoxification and rejuvenating program, or while one is concentrating on raising the urine pH back to normal (6.8 to 7.0).

Directions: Select and use a few organic vegetables from the moderate to strong alkaline vegetables listed on the previous pages, or as follows:

- Thick potato peelings (discard rest of potato)
- Carrot tops
- Beet tops
- Parsley
- Celery leaves and some stalk
- Other green vegetables, such as kelp, kale, etc.

Chop vegetables and place in a stainless steel pot with purified or filtered water. Bring to boil and simmer for 20 or 25 minutes. Let it cool a bit, then strain out the vegetable pieces, keeping the broth. As you are straining, squeeze the liquid out of the vegetable mass with a large spoon or potato masher to harvest all the mineral broth. Season the broth to taste with a vegetable salt such as Vegex, or Vege-Sal. Refrigerate and warm up portions as you consume it.

APPENDIX 8

RECIPES

The following recipes are presented as samples only. For more complete ideas, refer to other food preparation books written for healing with natural and organic foods.

Sprouted Seeds and Grains (Very healthy - full of enzymes and nutrients.)

Soak for 7 or 8 hours:

- 1 cup of organic rye grains
- 1 cup of organic barley grains
- 1 cup of organic sunflower seeds
- ¼ cup of organic sesame seeds

Rinse under cold water and drain well. Spread the drained grain and seeds on glass, non-ceramic plates, or sprouting dishes. Let sprout for 15 to 16 hours. During the time they are sprouting, rinse them under cool water at least twice or they will acquire a musty smell and taste. At the end of 16 hours, rinse well under cool water and strain. This mixture will last at least 3 days in the refrigerator.

To eat, mash a ripe raw banana in a bowl and add 1 or 2 tablespoons of natural strawberry jam. Add 1 cup or desired amount of sprouted seeds and grains and mix well.

Morning Pep Drink Meal

Soak overnight in the refrigerator:

- ¼ cup shelled, raw, unsalted, organic sunflower seeds
- 2 cups good water

In the morning, blend the seeds and water for 3 minutes at high speed. Add:

- 1-tablespoon brewers yeast
- 1-tablespoon blackstrap molasses
- 1-tablespoon acidophilus powder (or another probiotic product)

This is a full meal and should be sipped and chewed to mix well with saliva for proper digestion. For a more concentrated drink, double the quantity of sunflower seeds.

Vegetable Chop Suey

- 1-cup carrots, chopped
- 1-cup celery, chopped
- ½ cup green pepper, chopped
- ¼ to ½ red sweet pepper, chopped
- ½ cup onion, chopped (optional)
- 1-cup broccoli pieces
- ¼ lb. fresh mushrooms, whole or chopped
- 2 cups chicken stock
- 2 tablespoons tamari soy sauce or Braggs Liquid Aminos
- 2 tablespoons arrowroot powder or rice starch, tapioca starch, etc.
- 1 cup or more fresh bean sprouts

Add as desired -

- ½ teaspoon chopped fresh ginger
- 1 teaspoon chopped garlic
- 2 tablespoons black bean sauce

In a Chinese wok or heavy-bottom pot, stir-fry the vegetables (starting with the more solid ones first) in a liquid, such as water or chicken stock, until just tender but still crispy. Add chicken stock and tamari sauce and simmer, stirring constantly. (Seasoning, such as garlic or ginger, can be added to the stock beforehand to flavour to the stock.) Dissolve arrowroot powder in cold water, and add gradually, stirring until the mixture is cooked, and the liquid has thickened. Add raw bean sprouts just before serving. May be served with cooked brown rice.

Chicken Chop Suey
Same as above, but add 2 cups of cooked chicken cut in 1 inch pieces, at the same time as chicken stock is added. Since a protein has been added, it is best for proper food combining purposes to eat this meal without a carbohydrate, such as rice or bread.

Nut Milk
Good milk substitutes can be made in a blender using raw almonds, cashews, and sunflower or sesame seeds. Take one cup of good water and add about ¼ cup of raw nuts or seeds. Blend at high speed for 2 or 3 minutes, until thick white milk is formed. It is best used as it is, but it may also

be poured through sieve, gauze, or nutmilk bag to remove the pulp.

Hemp Seed Milk

Hemp seeds, being high in protein and essential fatty acids, make excellent pure white-coloured milk. Make it the same as Nut Milk above. Vary the amounts of water and hemp seeds according to your preference.

Simple Hemp Protein Drink

In a blender mix fruit, water and blend. Then add one or two tablespoons of hemp protein (rice protein is OK too). Blend again. Modify ingredients according to your taste. (Make sure that the protein powder you use has not been heat-processed.)

Hemp Protein Drink

Combine the following (or your own combination) in a blender, according to your taste. Blend, and add liquid as needed, as you proceed.

- 1 Cup or so of water or fresh juice
- 1 or 2 Tbs. Hemp seeds
- 1 Tbs. Hemp oil
- Apple and/or banana, strawberries, etc.
- 1 (or several) Tbs. Hemp protein powder
- 1 tsp. green super-food powder

<u>Optional</u>. Add one or more of the following:

- Flavouring, such as cinnamon or Oil of Orange
- ½ tsp. Powdered enzymes
- Rice protein powder
- Carob powder

This is very concentrated food. Eat it slowly, and mix it thoroughly with saliva in your mouth. This 'drink' contains everything to live on and build health in your body.

Protein Bars – These are terrific!

As with the Protein Drink, there are no hard and fast rules for making this concentrated, nutritious, meal and snack food. Use your own preferences and ideas regarding ingredients – be creative. Following, are the ingredients and procedures I usually use.

First, soak a cup of organic, whole, raw almonds and a cup of organic raw sunflower seeds in water overnight to activate enzymes. In the morning or later in the day when you are ready to make the bars, drain off the water and rinse each cup of nuts/seeds.

Second, in a good high speed blender, blend the following:
- ½ cup hemp oil
- 1 chopped apple (or other fruit)
- ½ cup unpasteurized honey
- Almonds (Add slowly, and work the mixture as it thickens)

Third, transfer this mixture into a large mixing bowl. When adding and mixing the following ingredients, I have found it easier to mix all ingredients, except the dry powders, with a large spoon. Then as I add the protein powders in, I work them into the mix by hand until I have achieved the desired consistency and dryness. (Wearing a pair of thin medical rubber gloves may help with clean-up.) (Using two sticks, such as chopsticks, to mix the ingredients thoroughly works very well too.)

Add the following one at a time and mix in thoroughly:

- Sunflower seeds
- ½ cup hemp seeds
- ½ cup sesame seeds
- 1 cup of finely chopped dried fruit (raisin, cherry, cranberry, currants, etc.)
- 1 cup or more hemp protein powder
- 1 or 2 Tbs. Green super-food powder

Optional. Add any of the following (you may think of others), to increase protein content and/or flavouring:

- Cinnamon
- Caraway seeds
- Oil of orange or lemon
- Fresh ground lemon rind
- Carob powder
- Rice protein powder

When you have the consistency (dryness/moisture content) to your liking, spoon out a large bar-sized amount of the mix onto a piece of waxed paper or plastic wrap. Or, form portions of the mix into small baseball size balls. Then place each one on a small sheet of clear plastic wrap. Fold the paper over and press down with a jar or rolling pin to the desired compactness and thickness. Square the bar and press again until you have the size and shape you want.

Store the bars in the fridge or freezer and eat them as you desire. However, they are very tasty and convenient so they probably won't stay there very long! This is complete, concentrated food that contains all the nutrition to sustain and grow a healthy body. Chew it thoroughly and eat it slowly. Enjoy.

Fruit Ice Cream

Use frozen raw bananas, strawberries, raspberries, or blueberries alone or in combination, and run through a Champion juicer with the solid screen cover in place. It tastes great and is nutritious because it still contains the natural enzymes and has no extra sugar or other additives.

Natural Strawberry Jam

- 2 cups of fresh or frozen strawberries (Can also use raspberries)
- 4 or 5 rings of dried pineapple
- Unsweetened pineapple or orange juice

Soak and rinse dried pineapple in water, to remove any sulphur. Cut dried pineapple into small pieces. Combine all ingredients and let set until dried pineapple is soft. Blend in blender until smooth. Juice may not need to be added if the strawberries have enough liquid. This is natural raw fruit. It is a good idea to put in small containers, and freeze any amount in excess of what you will use within a few days.

HOW TO USE A WATER ENEMA

The purpose of an enema is to efficiently and effectively clear the colon of toxic waste when the body is unable to do this adequately on its own. Enemas are recommended while fasting, undergoing an acute cleanse (healing crisis), during periods of detoxification for any serious or degenerative disease (can ease headaches at this time), or when there is a chronic constipation problem. Chemical laxatives are not the answer and should not be used.

Enemas are safe when used according to common sense instructions. The body does not become dependent on them when a person stops eating the toxic foods that caused the constipation problem in the first place, and begins to eat foods that will rebuild the body and restore health. In time, the colon will remove impacted fecal matter (the assistance of gentle herbs helps), slough off the old mucus coat, heal, and return to normal bowel function on its own. Taking enemas serves to help the body rid itself of toxins so that it can heal faster and exercise colon muscles. This tones them so that they can begin working efficiently on their own again.

Note: If the dietary habits that caused the colon problems are not discontinued, there will be no healing of the condition, and no matter what method is used to evacuate the colon – laxatives, or even enemas – these will appear to be habit forming. One must work to correct the cause of the problem.

INSTRUCTIONS:

1. Use a standard enema bag that can be purchased in most pharmacies. It should be able to hold 1 to 2 quarts or liters of water. The nozzle should be a regular nozzle, approximately 4 inches (10 centimeters) long.

2. Fill the enema bag with about a quart (or liter) for teenagers and adults. (Children would require one half or less this amount.) Use water that has been filtered to remove chlorine, fluorine, etc. The water should be of a temperature that is comfortable to the wrist. Slightly warmer (do not use hot) water can bring on more contractions, while cooler water has a toning effect on colon walls.

3. Hang the enema bag on a towel rack (or at that approximate height), using a bent coat hanger if a hook is not provided with the bag.

4. Lubricate the nozzle and rectum with K-Y gel, a vegetable oil, or an ordinary ointment. (Do not use Vaseline - it is a petroleum product.)

5. Kneel on the floor near the toilet, in the 'knee-chest' position so that the rectum is higher than the shoulders. This position allows for the water to run more easily

into the colon. If for some reason it is not possible to assume this position, lie on the right side or on the back. Alternatively, sit on the toilet so that leakage does not pose a clean-up problem

6. Insert the nozzle gently. If it will not go in all the way, it should do so once the flow of water is begun. It will be necessary to hold the nozzle in place with one hand throughout the enema session, as the body will tend to push it out.

7. Once the nozzle is in place, begin the flow of water from the enema bag into the colon. Regulate the flow of water into the colon so that it enters at a slow rate. Pinching or bending the hose does this. Most enema bags come with a flow regulator device.

8. As the water is flowing in, should any discomfort or an urge to expel the water be felt, stop the flow of water, take a few deep breaths and then resume the water flow as the urge passes.

9. Empty about 5 or 6 ounces of water from the enema bag into the colon. Should this be hindered because the urge to expel the water is too great, remove the enema nozzle, sit on the toilet, and expel whatever water is in the colon into the toilet. It should now be possible to resume the knee-chest position, and empty another 5 or 6 ounces of the water from the enema bag into the colon. If not, allow in what can comfortably be held in the colon.

10.   Once this water is in the colon, remove the nozzle from the rectum and lie on the floor resisting the urge to evacuate. Lie first on the left side, and then roll onto the back, then to the right side, then onto the stomach. Each position should be held for approximately 30 seconds. While lying on the back, the stomach/colon area can be gently massaged to promote better clearing of fecal matter. (Likewise, if you are doing the enema process while sitting on the toilet, you can massage your colon area with the other hand that is not holding the enema tip in place.)

11.   Next, sit on the toilet and expel the water. It may take several minutes for the water and contents to work their way out of the colon. One needs to be patient while waiting for the successive urges to evacuate.

12.   Should a good evacuation not be experienced, or not much water could be introduced into the colon, the enema bag can be immediately refilled and the entire process repeated. This may be done several times if necessary.

NOTE: This type of enema allows for a gentle release of toxins and built-up fecal matter from the lower end of the colon without stressing the body. It does not upset the over-all electrical balance of the colon or eliminate intestinal flora from the upper intestinal system.

PROBLEMS

Should the colon not be able to expel any or all of the water, introduce some water at a little warmer temperature into the colon, or slowly take another enema until some cramping and urge to evacuate begins. Likewise, should the colon be overactive, not allowing any or very little water to enter, use slightly cooler water. If only a small amount of water is able to enter into the colon, no more should be forced. Simply work with what will enter because it will be of benefit, providing it is stimulating a bowel movement.

In times of severe illness, enemas may not be sufficient. Colonics from a licensed colon therapist are much more effective and can be life-saving.

INDEX

Also available from
Crux Publishing

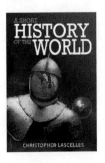

A Short History of the World
by Christopher Lascelles

'A clearly written, remarkably comprehensive guide to the greatest story on Earth - man's journey from the earliest times to the modern day. Highly recommended.'

DAN JONES, author of *The Plantagenets: The Kings Who Made England*

A Short History of the World is a short and easy-to-read history book that relates the history of our world from the Big Bang to the present day. It assumes no prior knowledge of past events and 32 maps have been especially drawn to give the reader a better understanding of where events occurred.

The book's purpose is not to come up with any ground-breaking new historical theories. Instead it aims to give a broad overview of the key events so that non-historians will feel less embarrassed about their lack of historical knowledge when discussing the past. The result is a history book that is reassuringly epic in scope but refreshingly short in length – an excellent place to start to bring your knowledge of world history up to scratch!

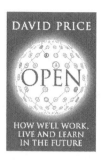

OPEN by David Price

'From every perspective OPEN will open your mind to some of the real implications of digital technologies for how we live and learn in the 21st century.'

SIR KEN ROBINSON,
world-leading expert on education and creativity

What makes a global corporation give away its prized intellectual property? Why are Ivy League universities allowing anyone to take their courses for free? What drives a farmer in rural Africa to share his secrets with his competitors?

A collection of hactivists, hobbyists, forum-users and maverick leaders are leading a quiet but unstoppable revolution. They are sharing everything they know, and turning knowledge into action in ways that were unimaginable even a decade ago. Driven by technology, and shaped by common values, going 'open' has transformed the way we live. It's not so much a question of if our workplaces, schools and colleges go open, but when.

Packed with illustration and advice, this entertaining read by learning futurist, David Price, argues that 'open' is not only affecting how we are choosing to live, but that it's going to be the difference between success and failure in the future.

Made in the USA
Charleston, SC
05 August 2014